Children and Exercise XXV

T0221379

The Proceedings of the 25th bi-annual Pediatric Work Physiology meeting present the most recent knowledge in the field of pediatric exercise sciences, focusing on the interaction between physical activity, exercise or sport on the one hand, and nutrition, metabolism regulation, cardiorespiratory function or muscle function on the other hand. The 44 chapters of this book are part of the 7 keynote lectures, 65 oral presentations and 66 poster presentations that were presented during the five day meeting. The book begins with chapters devoted to keynote lectures followed by shorter chapters arranged in 6 thematic sessions addressing:

- Metabolic syndrome and nutrition
- Hormonal and inflammatory regulations
- Cardiorespiratory functions
- Children's performances
- Fitness assessment
- Physical activity

Offering a critical review of current topic and reports and ongoing research in pediatric health and exercise science, this a key text for all researchers, teachers, health professionals and students with an interest in pediatric sport and exercise, sports medicine and physical education.

Georges Baquet is Senior Lecturer at the Faculty of Sports Sciences and Physical Education, University of Lille, France.

Serge Berthoin is Professor at the Faculty of Sports Sciences and Physical Education, University of Lille, France.

The Papers contained within this volume were first presented at the XXVth Pediatric Work Physiology meeting, held in Le Touquet, France, in September 2009.

Children and Exercise XXV

The proceedings of the 25th Pediatric Work
Physiology Meeting

Edited by

Georges Baquet and Serge Berthoin

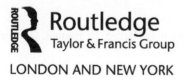

Routledge
Taylor & Francis Group

LONDON AND NEW YORK

This edition published 2011
by Routledge
2 Park Square, Milton Park, Abingdon, Oxon OX14 4RN

Simultaneously published in the USA and Canada
by Routledge
711 Third Avenue, New York, NY 10017

Routledge is an imprint of the Taylor & Francis Group, an informa business

First issued in paperback 2012

© 2011 Serge Berthoin and Georges Baquet

The right of the Author to be identified as author of this work has been asserted by him/her in accordance with sections 77 and 78 of the Copyright, Designs and Patents Act 1988.

Publisher's note
This book has been prepared from a camera-ready copy supplied by the authors

British Library Cataloguing in Publication Data
A catalogue record for this book is available from the British Library

Library of Congress Cataloging-in-Publication Data
Children and exercise XXV / edited by Serge Berthoin and Georges Baquet.

p. cm.

1. Exercise for children. 2. Physical fitness. I. Berthoin, Serge. II. Baquet, Georges.

GV443.C488 2011

613.7'042--dc22

2010015197

ISBN13: 978-0-415-57514-0 (hbk)
ISBN13: 978-0-415-68858-1 (pbk)
ISBN13: 978-0-203-85473-0 (ebk)

Contents

Part I

Keynote Lectures

Part II

Metabolic syndrome and nutrition

Part III

Hormonal and inflammatory regulations

Part IV

Cardiorespiratory functions

Part V

Children's performances

Part VI

Fitness assessment

Part VII

Physical activity

Preface

The XXVth Pediatric Work Physiology meeting was organized in Le Touquet, France, in September 2009. One hundred and thirty communications were presented as keynote lectures, oral or poster communications. As in the previous meetings during the last fifty years, all oral and poster presentations were presented in a unique auditorium maximizing possible exchanges between participants.

Symposium	Date	Place	Chair
I	1968	Dortmund, Germany	J. Rutenfranz
II	1969	Liblice, Czechoslovakia	V.S. Seliger
III	1970	Stockholm, Sweden	C. Thoren
IV	1972	Netanya, Israel	O. Bar-Or
V	1973	De Haan, Belgium	M. Hebbelinck
VI	1974	Sec, Czechoslovakia	M. Macek
VII	1975	Trois Rivières, Canada	R.J. Shephard
VIII	1976	Bisham, UK	C.T.M. Davies
IX	1978	Marstand, Sweden	B.O. Eriksson
X	1981	Jousta, Finland	J. Ilmarinen
XI	1983	Papendal, The Netherlands	R.A. Binkhorst
XII	1985	Hardehausen, Germany	J. Rutenfranz
XIII	1987	Hurdal, Norway	S. Oseid
XIV	1989	Leuven, Belgium	G. Beunen
XV	1989	Seregélyes, Hungary	R. Frenkl
XVI	1991	Saint-Sauves, France	J. Coudert, E. Van Praagh
XVII	1993	Hamilton, Canada	O. Bar-Or
XVIII	1995	Odense, Denmark	K. Froberg
XIX	1997	Exeter, UK	N. Armstrong
XX	1999	Sabaudia, Italy	A. Calzolari
XXI	2001	Corsendonk, Belgium	D. Matthys
XXII	2003	Porto, Portugal	J. Maia
XXIII	2005	Gwatt, Switzerland	S. Kriemler, N. Farpour-Lambert
XXIV	2007	Tallinn, Estonia	T. Jürimäe
XXV	2009	Le Touquet, France	G. Baquet, S. Berthoin

The meeting welcomes around 170 delegates coming from 22 countries including East and West Europe, North and South America, Asia, and Oceania.

The first part of the book begins with the 2009 Josef Rutenfranz lecture provided by Professor Emmanuel Van Praagh. A second chapter is dedicated to the memory of Professor Oded Bar-Or. This text is related to the tribute presented by Professor Han Kemper at the XXIVth Pediatric Work Physiology meeting that took place in 2007 in Tallinn, Estonia. The four remaining chapters of part I are related to the keynote lectures delivered by internationally renowned speakers.

The remaining chapters of the book are presented in six parts. They include four pages of communications mostly based on oral presentations.

Acknowledgments

International Scientific Committee

Pr Lars-Bo Andersen, University of Southern Denmark, Denmark
Pr Adam Baxter-Jones, University of Saskatchewan, Canada
Pr Ralph Beneke, University of Essex, United Kingdom
Dr Nathalie Boisseau, University of Poitiers, France
Pr Albrecht Claessens, Catholic University of Leuven, Belgium
Pr Daniel Courteix, Blaise Pascal University of Clermont-Ferrand, France
Pr Pascale Duché, Blaise Pascal University of Clermont-Ferrand, France
Pr Ulf Ekelund, Cambridge University, United Kingdom
Pr Helge Hebestreit, University of Würzburg, Germany
Pr Régis Matran, University of Lille 2, France
Pr Philippe Obert, University of Avignon, France
Pr Jean-Michel Oppert, Pierre and Marie Curie University-Paris 6, France
Pr Jacques Poortmans, Free University of Bruxelles, Belgium
Pr Gareth Stratton, John Moores University, Liverpool, United Kingdom
Pr Mark Tremblay, University of Ottawa, Canada
Pr Jos Twisk, Free University of Amsterdam, The Netherlands
Pr Willem van Mechelen, Free University of Amsterdam, The Netherlands
Pr Craig Williams, University of Exeter, United Kingdom

Acknowledgments

International Organizing Committee

Pr Neil Armstrong, University of Exeter, United Kingdom
Dr Georges Baquet, University of Lille 2, France
Pr Serge Berthoin, University of Lille 2, France
Pr Gaston Beunen, Catholic University of Leuven, Belgium
Pr Nathalie Farpour-Lambert, Geneve University Hospital, Switzerland
Pr Karsten Froberg, University of Southern Denmark, Denmark
Pr Frédéric Gottrand, University of Lille 2, France
Pr Toivo Jürimäe, University of Tartu, Estonia
Pr Han CG Kemper, Free University of Amsterdam, The Netherlands
Pr Susi Kriemler, University of Zurich, Switzerland
Pr Jose Maïa, University of Porto, Portugal
Pr Thomas Rowland, Baystate Medical Center, Springfield, United States
Pr Viswanath Unnithan, Liverpool Hope University, United Kingdom
Pr Emmanuel Van Praagh, Blaise Pascal University, Clermont-Ferrand, France

Acknowledgments

Local Organizing Committee

Georges Baquet
Serge Berthoin
Anne Sophie Bierinx
Mickael Bisiaux
Aurélie Blaes
Julien Boissière
Benoit Borel
Valérie Bougault
Isabelle Caby
Patricia Demerlier
Claudine Fabre
François-Xavier Gamelin
Yasmine Guemra
Elsa Heyman
Erwan Leclair
Ghislaine Lensel
Patrick Mucci
Mathieu Nédélec
Nicolas Voy

And a big thank-you to **Jean-Marie Deruelle** for his valuable help

Acknowledgments

Sponsors

Lille 2, Law and Health University, France
Faculty of Sports Sciences and Physical Education, Lille, France
Nord-Pas de Calais Regional Council, France
Pas de Calais Department Council, France
Le Touquet Paris-Plage, France
Faber France, Wexilum, France
TSP Diffusion, France

Part I

Keynote Lectures

The 2009 Josef Rutenfranz Lecture "Child as a Source of Mechanical Power"

E. Van Praagh

Blaise Pascal University, Clermont-Ferrand, France

1.1 INTRODUCTION

Since the early aerobic fitness studies conducted by S. Robinson (1938) on males aged 6 to 91 and P.O. Astrand (1952) on both females and males aged 4 to 33, more recent work done by pediatric exercise scientists were very comparable to these initial studies. Tomkinson and Olds (2007) showed that there has been a decline in pediatric aerobic performance since 1970, a pattern which is not observed in pediatric anaerobic performance. The following questions will be addressed: Is there evidence of an age-related decline in physical activity (PA)? Are children more motivated by short-term high intensity exercise than long-term low intensity exercise? How to measure short-term bouts of exercise during growth? What are the main biological determinants?

1.2 AGE-RELATED DECLINE IN PHYSICAL ACTIVITY?

Several studies have demonstrated a decline of PA in children (Sallis, 2000). It is commonly believed that boys are more physically active than girls. Nyberg *et al.* (2009) reported that this decline may start already at the age of 6 yr. Thompson *et al.* (2003) showed if PA decreased with increasing chronological age in boys and girls, there were no gender differences in the longitudinal pattern of PA when the confounding effects of biological age were controlled. More recently Sherar *et al.* (2007) confirmed that to fully understand gender disparities in PA, consideration must be given to the confounding effects of physical maturity.

1.3 SHORT-TERM EXERCISE OR LONG-TERM EXERCISE?

Most of the scientific pediatric literature is devoted to the study of prolonged maximal power output (Baquet *et al.*, 2003), but comparatively little attention has been given to maximal intensity exercise lasting only a few seconds. This is surprising, considering that in almost all daily tasks, games in the playground or multiple sprint sports (such as team ball games, racket sports, sprint- and running events), the child is primarily more involved in short-term high-intensity exercise (HIE) than in long-term activities. Already in 1938, Sid Robinson noted after a strenuous $\dot{V}O_2$ max test: "the fact that the younger boys do not produce higher lactates may depend on an *unwillingness* to continue work after it ceases to *entertain* them". Showing that PA is not only directed by biological factors, but that psychological factors such as motivation have also an important role during the development period. Reporting that many problems persist in the accurate assessment of energy expenditure, especially in non-laboratory settings under natural conditions, Bailey *et al.* (1995) developed a direct *observational* approach for quantifying patterns of frequency, duration, and intensity of PA. The most striking outcome was the short duration of activity events, especially those in the high-intensity range. Recent data showed that, using high-frequency accelerometry during a 7-days PA assessment in prepubertal girls and boys, ninety-six percent of very-high physical activity (VHPA) presented a duration of less than 10 s. (Baquet *et al.*, 2007). Moreover, it was also recently shown that the main component of activity that differs between girls and boys and between high- and low-active children is the frequency of the most intense bouts (Rowlands *et al.*, 2008).

1.4   HOW TO MEASURE 'ANEROBIC FITNESS' DURING GROWTH?

1.4.1   Invasive methods

The first studies using the needle biopsy technique in the pediatric population were done in the US (Brooke and Engel, 1969) and in Sweden (Eriksson *et al.*, 1971). Muscle tissue was obtained during surgical intervention (trauma or orthopaedic operations). Few studies on muscle storage of phosphagens have shown that the content of the peripheral energy-delivering substrates is the same for both children and adults. In several textbooks and scientific reports, it is still assumed that the rate of anaerobic glycolysis is limited in children because of their lower phospho-fructokinase (PFK) activity. However, this assumption is only discussed on the basis of the results of PFK at rest (Eriksson *et al.*, 1971). It is interesting that during some 30 years, it was speculated that the lower glycolytic ability during short-term HIE of the child (e.g. lower lactate values, lower short-term power outputs) was due to lower glycogen content and glycolytic enzyme activities at rest. Within the limited available evidence from muscle biopsy studies, it seems necessary to consider other metabolic factors than only the muscle enzyme activities at rest or post-exercise.

1.4.2   Non-invasive method: 31P-NMRS

The first NMR study of muscle bioenergetics during exercise was reported by E. Purcell and F. Bloch (1946). Both won the Nobel Prize in Physics in 1952 (for review, Sapega *et al.*, 1987). In children, the use of nuclear magnetic resonance spectroscopy (NMRS) now provides a safe and non-invasive means of monitoring intracellular inorganic phosphate [Pi], PCr, ATP and pH at rest, during exercise and recovery (Cooper and Barstow, 1996). Zanconato *et al.* (1993) established the profiles of Pi/PCr and pH in the calf muscle of children and adults performing, at the same intensity, a progressive (plantar flexion) exercise. The minimal drop in pH seen in children and the fact that they achieved an end-exercise Pi/PCr value of only 27% of adult values, are consistent with several reports of the relatively low muscle and blood lactate responses to short-term HIE in children. During short-term HIE and recovery, intramuscular high-energy phosphate kinetics is attenuated in children compared with adults. Although NMRS has proved to be a unique tool for investigating muscle metabolism during exercise, 'progressive plantar flexion' may be a poor representation of whole body anaerobic responses.

1.4.3 Wilkie's statement

During childhood and adolescence, direct measurements of the rate or capacity of anaerobic pathways for energy turnover presents several ethical and methodological difficulties. To quote Wilkie (1960), "In children, exercise scientists instead of attempting to quantify anaerobic energy yield by ATP or glycolysis, are more inspired to measure the resulting mechanical output during short-term exercise, which is the truly useful product".

This statement makes the assessment of anaerobic performance more "powerful", since only the subject's maximal performance will be considered as the criterion. Therefore, during growth, the measurement of mechanical output during short-term high-intensity exercise is a reasonable and useful alternative for elaborating innovative techniques and procedures.

1.4.4 Short-term mechanical power output during growth

Assessment of short-term power raises several methodological problems: (for review see Van Praagh and Doré, 2002).

1. Since power is the product of force and velocity, the external load (e.g. body mass during jumping or load on the cycle ergometer) must closely match the capability of the active muscles so that they operate at their optimal velocity (Wilkie, 1960). Clearly, this is a difficult condition to fulfil or to guarantee in freely accelerating or decelerating cycling or running sprint efforts. Several activities have been proposed for the measurement of short-term power output, including vertical jumping, running or cycling. Of these activities, only cycle ergometry allows precise measurement of power independent of body mass as the imposed load.

2. If 'true' short-term peak power output (STPPO) is to be measured, the duration of the test must be as short as possible, because power output decreases rapidly as a function of time (Wilkie, 1960; Van Praagh *et al.*, 1991). The measurement of "true" STPPO requires measurements of instantaneous values of force and velocity.

3. Anaerobic glycolysis and aerobic contribution are limited during instantaneous power tests, although the aerobic fraction in young people is higher than in young men (Van Praagh *et al.*, 1991; Beneke *et al.*, 2007). According to Ferretti *et al.* (1994) only exercises lasting a few seconds can be considered as truly 'alactacid'.

1.5   WHAT ARE THE MAIN BIOLOGICAL DETERMINANTS?

STPPO and 'anaerobic fitness' are quantitative traits influenced by several factors such as age, gender and training. However, STPO is also determined by innate biological and mechanical variables. Although age – and gender-related differences in the adaptive response to STPO might be related to the maturation of muscle metabolism pathways, little is known about the underlying mechanisms. Differences found between children and young adults during STPPO testing are mainly attributed to size-dependent factors (e.g. muscle size) and size-independent factors (e.g. genetics, hormonal factors). Although in progress, little attention has been devoted to understanding the biological basis of physical activity (Rowland, 1998). However, more and more candidate genes are now being identified and it is clear that heredity contributes to the physical activity phenotype (Eisenmann and Wickel, 2009).

1.6   CONCLUSION

Considering that children are spontaneously more involved in short-burst activities than in long-term low-intensity exercises, short-term peak power output (STPPO) is a fundamental aspect of the child's physical capacity. There is a general agreement that STPPO increases during growth and maturation and is significantly higher in boys than in girls during and after the adolescent growth spurt. However, in this particular pediatric exercise science area, there has been much relevant applied research, but there is a need for more fundamental research to obtain further knowledge regarding the underlying mechanisms implied in short-term high-intensity physical activity.

1.7   REFERENCES

Åstrand, P.O., 1952, Experimental studies of the physical working capacity in relation to sex and age. Copenhagen, Munksgaar.

Bailey, R.C., Olson, J., Pepper, S.J., Porszasz, J., Barstow, T.J. and Cooper, D.M., 1995, The level and tempo of children's physical activities: an observational study. *Medicine and Science in Sports and Exercise,* **27**, pp. 1033–1041.

Baquet, G., Van Praagh, E. and Berthoin, S., 2003, Endurance training and aerobic fitness in young people. *Sports Medicine*, **33**, pp. 1127–1143.

Baquet, G., Stratton, G., Van Praagh, E. and Berthoin, S., 2007, Improving physical activity assessment in prepubertal children with high-frequency accelerometry monitoring: A methodological issue. *Preventive Medicine*, **44**, pp. 143–147.

Beneke, R., Hütler, M. and Leithäuser, R.M., 2007, Anaerobic performance and metabolism in boys and male adolescents. *European Journal of Applied Physiology*, **101**, pp. 671-677.

Brooke, M.H. and Engel, W.K., 1969, The histographic analysis of human muscle biopsies with regard to fibre types: children's biopsies. *Neurology*, **19**, pp. 591–605.

Cooper, D.M. and Barstow, T.J., 1996, Magnetic resonance imaging and spectroscopy in studying exercise in children; in Holloszy JO (ed): *Exercise and Sports Science Reviews.* Baltimore, Williams and Wilkins, pp. 475–499.

Eisenmann, J.C. and Wickel, E.E., 2009, The biological basis of physical activity in children: revisited. *Pediatric Exercise Science*, **21**, pp. 257–272.

Eriksson, B.O., Karlsson, J. and Saltin, B., 1971, Muscle metabolites during exercise in pubertal boys. *Acta Paediatrica Scandinavica*, **217**, pp. S154–S157.

Ferreti, G., Narici, M.V., Binzoni, T., Gariod, L., Le Bas, J.F., Reutenauer, H. and Cerretelli, P., 1994, Determinants of peak muscle power: effects of age and physical conditioning. *European Journal of Applied Physiology*, **68**, pp. 111–115.

Nyberg, G.A., Nordenfelt, A.M., Ekelund, U. and Marcus, C., 2009, Physical activity patterns measured by accelerometry in 6-to-10-yr-old children. *Medicine and Science in Sports and Exercise*, **41**, pp. 1842–1848.

Robinson, S., 1938, Experimental studies of physical fitness in relation to age. *Arbeitsphysiologie*, **10**, pp. 251–323.

Rowland, T.W., 1998, The biological basis of physical activity. *Medicine and Science in Sports and Exercise*, **30**, pp. 392–399.

Rowlands, A.V., Pilgrim, E.L. and Eston, R.G., 2008, Patterns of habitual activity across weekdays and weekend days in 9-11 year-old children. *Preventive Medicine*, **46**, pp. 317–324.

Sallis, J.F., 2000, Age-related decline in physical activity: a synthesis of human and animal studies. *Medicine and Science in Sports and Exercise*, **32**, pp. 1598–1600.

Sapega, A.A., Sokolow, D.P., Graham, T.J. and Chance, B., 1987, Phosphorus nuclear magnetic resonance: a non–invasive technique for the study of muscle bioenergetics during exercise. *Medicine and Science in Sports and Exercise*, **19**, pp. 410–420.

Sherar, L.B., Esliger, D.W., Baxter-Jones, A.D. and Tremblay, M.S., 2007, Age and gender differences in youth physical activity: does physical maturity matter? *Medicine and Science in Sports and Exercise*, **39**, pp. 830–835.

Thompson, A.M., Baxter-Jones, A., Mirwald, R.L. and Bailey, D.A., 2003, Comparison of physical activity in male and female children: does maturation matter? *Medicine and Science in Sports and Exercise*, **35**, pp. 1684–1690.

Tomkinson, G.R., and Olds, T.S., 2007, Secular changes in pediatric aerobic fitness test performance: the global picture. In *Pediatric Fitness, Secular Trends and Geographic Variability.* Medicine and Sport Science. (Karger, Basel), vol. **50**, pp.46–66.

Van Praagh, E., Bedu, M., Falgairette, G., Fellmann, N. and Coudert, J., 1991, Oxygen uptake during a 30-s supramaximal exercise in 7-to-15-year-old boys; in Frenkl R, Smodis I (eds): *Children and Exercise: Pediatric Work Physiology.* Budapest, National Institute for Health Promotion, pp. 281–287.

Van Praagh, E. and Doré, E., 2002, Short-term muscle power during growth and maturation. *Sports Medicine*, **32**, pp. 701–728.

Wilkie, D.R., 1960, Man as a source of mechanical power. *Ergonomics*, **3**, pp. 1–8.

Zanconato, S., Buchtal, S., Barstow, T.J. and Cooper, D.M., 1993, 31P-magnetic resonance spectroscopy of leg muscle metabolism during exercise in children and adults. *Journal of Applied Physiology*, **74**, pp. 2214–2218.

Oded Bar-Or (1936-2005) "Father"of the European Group of Paediatric Work Physiology: Children and Exercise

H.C.G. Kemper

Emeritus Professor in Health and Activity, VU University Medical Center,
EMGO+ Institute for preventive care and health, The Netherlands

This paper summarizes the importance of Oded Bar-Or for the European group of paediatric work physiology (PWP) that organized international symposia from 1968 till the present, about children and exercise.

2.1   THE LAST TIME

The last time I met Oded was on Sunday the 25th of September 2005. It was during the 23rd meeting of the European group of Pediatric Work Physiology (in short: PWPXXIII) in Gwatt (Switzerland). At that conference, although fatigued from his illness and in considerable discomfort, he courageously presented a keynote address titled "Energy Cost of Locomotion in Paediatric Health and Disease".

After the discussion of his talk, I was asked to say some words to Oded on behalf of all the participants, because we sadly realized that this PWP conference would probably be his last, and this was most likely the final lecture of his that we would hear. His wife, Marilyn, was there during the whole conference, and it was wonderful to see that Oded did his utmost to present an excellent lecture for us. In a few words I tried to express the importance of Oded's work for the advancement of scientific knowledge about physiological principles and clinical applications for children and exercise. It appeared to be his final presentation of many papers and keynotes in former PWP meetings (Farpour-Lambert *et al.*, 2005).

2.2   THE FIRST TIME

It was in Natanya, Israel, where I met Oded for the first time in April 1972. He was on the organizing committee of the PWP IV conference and was also the editor of the proceedings (Bar-Or, 1973). For me as a young scientist, it was my first attendance in this group of exercise physiologists, paediatricians, cardiologists and physical educators. Oded was everywhere as organizer, as lecturer (four presentations) and always actively participating in the discussions with such experienced participants as Joseph Rutenfranz, Bengt Eriksson, Roy Shephard, Simon Godfrey, Rolf Mocellin and Gordon Cumming.

For me it was a step forward in exercise science, not only because of the quality of most of the presentations but most of all because of the discussions that occurred without regard to prestige and always supporting the presented research.

I also met his wife Marilyn and their three small children in their home on the campus of Wingate Institute and I was impressed by the cellar that led down to their private underground shelter for air-raid bombing attacks from neighbouring countries (the war ended in 1967).

I was surprised when Oded and his co-workers Zwiren (1973) and Weingarten (1973) presented papers (about the effects of increased frequency and content variation of physical education classes in 9-10 year-old girls and boys, since I had just published comparable randomized control trials in 12-13 year-old boys in the Netherlands (Kemper *et al.*, 1971; Kemper, 1973).

2.3   ODED ON THE MOVE

Since then we met each other at almost all PWP conferences that took place every other year - in total twenty times, not taking into account his visits to our University in Amsterdam during his visiting professorship in 1989 at Maastricht, University of Limbourg in the Netherlands and at other international conferences such as the annual meetings of the ACSM in the United States.

It was Oded's initiative also to organize a "European" PWP conference outside Europe in 1977 in Trois Rivières in Canada.

In Canada (Hamilton at McMaster University) he wrote his outstanding book *Pediatric Sports Medicine for the Practitioner: from physiologic principles to clinical applications*, published in 1983 (Bar-Or, 1983) and lectured about it in several PWP conferences. As keynote lecturer he proved to be a gifted speaker who inspired many young investigators.

After the early death in 1988 of Joseph Rutenfranz (Dortmund, Germany) -- one of the founder members of the PWP -- Oded gave in 1995 the Rutenfranz lecture at PWP XVIII in Odense (Denmark) about "safe exercise for the child with chronic disease" (Bar-Or, 1997).

In 1991 we had our PWP XVI in Saint Sauves in France and because Oded was a frequent flyer, giving papers and advice all over the world, sometimes he got into trouble arriving late or departing early because of other obligations.

In St Sauves Oded and I were asked to decide the Young Investigator awards for the best presentation and poster. The organizing committee planned the announcement to be made during the last dinner. Half an hour before the start of the ceremony Oded came to me in his tracksuit, in panic, asking for some decent clothes for him to wear. He had given all his dirty ones to be washed, but they had not yet arrived and the hotel management expected them only the next morning. So we went to my room to see which jacket, shirt, trousers and tie should fit. He took them with him and just before dinner he arrived nicely dressed but (as he laughingly whispered in my ear) without any underwear!

2.4 "FATHER" OF PWP

If Joseph Rutenfranz can be characterized as the founding "grandfather" of the PWP conferences, Oded can be labelled as the "father" of these PWP (Figure 2.1). He always stressed the importance of holding symposia at venues outside big cities, with no parallel sessions; and he started a novelty and trend in 1983 (at the PWPXI conference in Papendal, The Netherlands) with scheduling poster sessions: They were grouped together on different topics and scheduled in the program with discussions about each poster after a two or three minute presentation by the author.

But Oded was also North American and in the 1980s he was also involved in the formation of the North American Society of Pediatric Exercise Medicine (NASPEM).

This group also started to organize their own conferences. Oded took the initiative to have a combined PWP/NASPEM conference. It showed his straddle position between PWP and NASPEM.

Together with Joe Blimkie, and with Marilyn and their daughter Tali Bar-Or as members in the organizing committee, a combined meeting (PWP XVII) was organized in 1993 in Hamilton, Ontario, Canada and resulted in a well known publication "New Horizons in Pediatric Exercise Science" edited by Joe Blimkie and Oded Bar-Or (Blimkie *et al.*, 1995). This title expresses exactly what Oded preached in his research: always be in the forefront of exercise and children's health.

At the PWP XXII in Porto (Portugal in 2003) Claude Bouchard presented a lecture for Oded Bar-Or at his official retirement, although nobody believed that he would retire from his hobby: research in children and exercise.

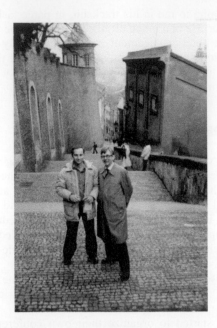

Figure 2.1. "Grandfather" Joseph Rutenfranz (right) and "father" Oded Bar-Or (left) together at one of the former PWP conferences in Prague (then Czechoslovakia).

2.5   WITHOUT ODED

On March 26, 2004 Oded was present in Amsterdam at the symposium that was organized by my colleagues van Mechelen and Twisk for my own retirement.

From the Brock University in Canada he received in the beginning of 2005 an honorary degree and during my visit in April 2005 at the Brock University with John Hay, I spoke to Oded on the phone but he was too tired to meet for a barbecue.

In December 8 that same year he died.

Two years later at the XXIVth PWP meeting in Tallinn (Estonia) the organizers decided to pay a special session to Oded. Bareket Falk, Emanuel van Praagh and I were invited to memorialize (or use 'recall') his life, his work and his leadership.

Oded will be remembered by all members of the European Group of Paediatric Work Physiology as an excellent scientist and gifted lecturer. Although we will never see him, never speak with him or never listen to him anymore, his outstanding scientific work can still always be read from his numerous published articles in journals, abstracts in conference proceedings, and (chapters in) books.

Oded Bar-Or's spirit for research in exercise for children's health will be continued in memorial lectures in future PWP meetings, as realized for the first time in the XXIVth PWP organized in Laulasmaa (Tallinn, Estonia) in 2007, and also at the XXVth conference in Le Touquet (France) in 2009.

2.6 REFERENCES

Part of this presentation was published earlier in Paediatric Exercise Science Memorial Issue Oded Bar-Or 1936-2005, *Pediatric Exercise Science*, 2006, **18**, pp.155–157.

Bar-Or, O. (ed.), 1973, Pediatric Work Physiology, Proceedings of the Fourth International Symposium, Wingate Institute, Natanya, Israel.

Bar-Or, O., 1983, *Pediatric Sports Medicine for the Practitioner, From Physiologic Principles to Clinical Applications*, Springer-Verlag, New York.

Bar-Or, O., 1997, Safe exercise for the child with a chronic disease. In: *Exercise and Fitness- benefits and risks*, K. Froberg, O. Lammert, H. St Hansen, C.J.R. Blimkie (eds) Children and Exercise XVIII, Odense University Press, Odense, pp. 15–27.

Bar-Or, O, 2005, Energy cost of locomotion in paediatric health and disease. In: Children and Exercise XXIII (Farpour-Lambert, N, Stüssi, Ch, Kriemler, S. eds). Gwatt, Switzerland, Part 6, pp. 49–51.

Blimkie, C.J.R. and Bar-Or, O., 1995, *New Horizons in Pediatric Exercise Science*. Human Kinetics, Champaign, IL.

Farpour-Lambert, N., Stüssi, C. and Kriemler, S. (eds.), 2005, Proceedings of the XXIII International Meeting of the European Group of Pediatric Work Physiology, Gwatt, Switzerland.

Kemper, H.C.G., Poulus, A.J. and van der Helm, N., 1971, Training und Körpererziehung: Über den Einfluss einer Kreistrainings beim Schulsport auf einige morphologische und funktionelle Merkmale bei 12-13jährigen Jungen. *Medizin und Sport*, **6**, pp. 179–184.

Kemper, H.C.G., 1973, The influence of extra lessons in physical education on physical and mental development of 12- and 13-year-old boys, In: Seliger, V. (ed.) *Physical Fitness*, Universita Kurlova, Prague, pp. 212–216.

Weingarten, G. and Bar-Or, O., 1973, The effects of frequency and content variation of physical education classes on social and athletic status in 4th grade children. In: Bar-Or, O. (editor) Pediatric Work Physiology, proceedings of the fourth international symposium, Wingate Institute for Sport and Physical Education Authority in the Ministry of Education and Culture, Tel-Aviv, Israel, pp. 199–207.

Zwiren, L.D. and Bar- Or, O., 1973, Physiological effects of increased frequency of physical education classes end of endurance conditioning on 9 to 10 year-old girls and boys. In: Bar-Or, O. (Ed) Pediatric Work Physiology, proceedings of the fourth international symposium, Wingate Institute for Sport and Physical Education Authority in the Ministry of Education and Culture, Tel-Aviv, Israel, pp. 183–199.

Obesity and Cardiovascular Function in Children and Adolescents

D.J. Green

Research Institute for Sport and Exercise Science, Liverpool John Moores University, School of Sports Science, Exercise, UK and Health, The University of Western Australia, Australia

3.1 ATHEROSCLEROSIS AS A DISEASE OF CHILDHOOD AND THE IMPORTANCE OF PREVENTION

There is now broad acceptance that the prevalence of overweight/obesity, insulin resistance and type 2 diabetes is increasing in highly urbanised western countries and, in particular, in lower socioeconomic postal ("zip") codes. There are also data emerging from China and India, populous countries with a burgeoning "middle-class", which suggest very large increases in the levels of childhood and adolescent obesity and diabetes. These data have led to some dire predictions. For example, a Special Report published in the New England Journal of Medicine concluded that: "Unless population-level interventions to reduce obesity are developed, the steady rise in life expectancy observed in the modern era may soon come to an end and the youth of today may, on average, live less healthy and possibly even shorter lives than their parents" (Olshansky *et al.*, 2005).

It is fair to say that, because clinical manifestations typically emerge in latter decades of life, atherosclerosis has traditionally been perceived as a disease of older people. However, evidence derived from autopsy studies performed in US personnel who died in the Korean war indicated that ~80% of 22 year olds had some evidence of coronary atherosclerosis. A more recent study endorsed this proportion and added that 20% of relatively young individuals (mean 26 yrs) had >50%, and ~10% had >75%, coronary stenoses. Intravascular ultrasound studies also suggest that atherosclerosis begins at a young age and other studies have reported that neonates who are small for their gestational age exhibit aortic thickening, suggesting a role for foetal programming in atherogenesis. Taken together, these data suggest that atherosclerosis begins early in life and that preventative measures should be focussed on young subjects who are at elevated risk.

3.2 ATHEROSCLEROSIS AND ENDOTHELIAL DYSFUNCTION IN CHILDHOOD AND ADOLESCENCE

The findings above raise the issue of identifying young asymptomatic individuals who are at the highest risk of future disease manifestation. Despite decades of development and refinement, algorithms based on traditional risk factors fail to predict cardiovascular disease in 25-50% of cases (Naghavi *et al.*, 2003). Indeed, a recent American Heart Association expert review concluded that high Framingham scores fall short in providing a clear clinical route for identification of future victims of acute coronary syndromes and sudden cardiac death (Naghavi *et al.*, 2003). Framingham and NCEP risk scores also fail to reflect the amount of atherosclerotic disease detected by CT. One reason for this risk factor prediction "gap" is that the majority of cardiovascular events are due to plaque rupture and the factors which predispose to rupture are not identical to those which predict atherosclerotic development.

Assessment of endothelial dysfunction in humans represents an attractive CV risk prediction candidate, as it is associated with plaque vulnerability, thrombogenesis and reflects the compound impact of traditional cardiovascular risk factors on atherogenic development. Endothelial dysfunction is now recognised as an early manifestation of atherosclerotic disease and some evidence suggests that it is a causal event, rather than merely an "epiphenomenon". Flow mediated dilation (FMD), a non-invasive assessment of nitric oxide (NO)-mediated endothelial function, provides independent prognostic information which exceeds that available from traditional risk factors in asymptomatic subjects and those with existing cardiovascular disease. FMD also predicts the progression of structural atherosclerotic change in the arterial wall. Taken together, these findings suggest that early detection and treatment of endothelial dysfunction may represent a novel primary prevention strategy in adolescents who are at elevated risk for development of cardiovascular disease in later life.

Studies dating back to 1992 indicate that children and adolescents at risk of atherosclerosis demonstrate endothelial dysfunction. Cigarette smoking, passive smoking and familial hypercholesterolaemia are all associated with endothelial dysfunction in young people. More recently, we (Watts *et al.*, 2004a; Watts *et al.*, 2004b) and others completed studies in which endothelial function in children and adolescents with obesity was impaired relative to age and gender matched lean controls, suggesting the presence of early atherogenic changes in both groups (Figure 3.1). These data were confirmed by finding in obese children that endothelial dysfunction was related to indices of insulin resistance, suggesting that endothelial dysfunction may be an antecedent of type 2 diabetes and the metabolic syndrome in obese children. We have previously demonstrated that endothelial function was impaired in adults with type 2 diabetic subjects (Maiorana *et al.*, 2001; Maiorana *et al.*, 2002*)*.

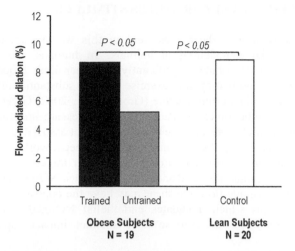

Figure 3.1 Endothelium-dependent, flow-mediated dilation (FMD) of the brachial artery in lean control subjects, and in obese adolescent subjects following a randomised cross-over trial of the effects of inactivity and exercise training. FMD, a largely nitric oxide (NO)-mediated endothelium-dependent phenomenon (Joannides *et al.*, 1995) is impaired in the presence of obesity. These data indicate that obese children and adolescents exhibit an early manifestation of atherosclerosis. Exercise training was associated with a normalisation of the FMD response.

3.3 CAN ENDOTHELIAL FUNCTION BE IMPROVED? WHAT IS THE PHYSIOLOGICAL STIMULUS TO ENHANCED ENDOTHELIAL FUNCTION?

It has been well documented since the 1930s that acute changes in blood flow signal flow-induced dilation of arteries in animals. In the 1980's the landmark work of Rubanyi *et al.* demonstrated that increases in blood flow rate through the lumen of arteries, and hence wall shear stress, leads to arterial dilation, transduced by a substance (or substances) released from endothelium. Pohl *et al.* simultaneously discovered that vasomotor responses to increased flow are critically dependent upon an intact and functional endothelial lining, suggesting that endothelial cells act as mediators of NO-dependent flow-mediated dilation (FMD). We recently confirmed this work in humans by demonstrating that arteries denuded of an endothelial lining demonstrated impaired FMD in response to a flow or shear stress stimulus.

In addition to the impact of shear forces on endothelial function, it is now well established that change in the circumferential size of arteries, "arterial remodelling", is also dependent upon shear stress, transduced through a functional endothelium. Hence, artery function, remodelling and wall morphology (eg thickness, stiffness) are all dependent upon, and modulated by, the endothelium. Acute and chronic changes in blood flow, and shear forces, induce adaptation in artery function and structure which are transduced by the endothelium.

3.4   EXERCISE AS A SHEAR STRESS STIMULUS

Exercise increases arterial shear stress and in this way modulates endothelial function and arterial remodelling in animals. In humans, we observed that endothelial function contributes significantly to upper limb blood flow during lower limb exercise and that cycling exercise induces substantial retrograde flows through the upper limbs during diastole (Green *et al.*, 2002; Green *et al.*, 2004). This effect appears to be driven by changes in pulse pressure since increasing pulse rate in the absence of changes in pulse pressure was not associated with changes in endothelial function. These observations have led to recent work characterising the impact of different forms of exercise on arterial shear forces and the observation that increases in antegrade flow and shear stress enhance NO-mediated endothelial function, whilst retrograde flow and shear may have the opposite impact. Exercise is clearly a stimulus which modulates endothelial NO-mediated function, but different types or forms of exercise have distinct impacts upon endothelial function.

3.5   EFFECTS OF EXERCISE TRAINING ON ENDOTHELIAL FUNCTION

Exercise training improves NO-mediated responses (Green *et al.*, 2004) and upregulates NO-synthase expression in animals. We have reported improved indices of arterial remodelling in humans, as well as enhanced endothelium-dependent NO function in patients with heart failure, coronary disease and hypercholesterolaemia. We also provided the first evidence that exercise training improves endothelial function in adults with type 2 diabetic subjects (Maiorana *et al.*, 2001; Maiorana *et al.*, 2002). These data suggest that exercise training may have important clinical significance in diabetes, since improvement in endothelial function parallels anti-atherogenic benefits and may ameliorate the vascular complications which account for most deaths in type 2 diabetic subjects.

    To assess inter-relationships between exercise training-mediated changes in artery function and remodelling we recently studied brachial and popliteal artery function and structure every 2 weeks across an 8-week exercise program in healthy young men (Tinken *et al.*, 2008). Vascular function adapted rapidly to training, whilst arterial size increased toward the end of the training period as function returned to baseline levels. These results support the notion, initially advanced by Laughlin and colleagues, that shear stress mediated arterial remodelling, which is at least partly NO-dependent, acts to mitigate the increases in shear stress brought about by repeated exercise bouts.

    Finally, we recently studied the role of shear stress in transducing changes associated with exercise training (Tinken *et al.*, 2009). Bilateral hand-grip exercise of matching intensity and duration was undertaken in both arms, with an inflated cuff around one forearm to attenuate the increase in blood flow and shear stress during each exercise bout, relative to the contralateral limb. Whilst changes in FMD and evidence for both conduit and resistance artery remodelling were observed in the limb exposed to episodic increases in blood flow and shear, no changes in artery function or structure were apparent in the contralateral limb in which flow/shear changes had been controlled. These data are the first to have directly manipulated shear stress during exercise training and observed differences in arterial adaptation in humans.

3.6 EFFECTS OF EXERCISE TRAINING ON ENDOTHELIAL FUNCTION IN CHILDREN AND ADOLESCENTS

We (Watts *et al.*, 2004a; Watts *et al.*, 2004b) and others have demonstrated that exercise training enhances endothelial function (FMD) in obese children and adolescents (Figure 3.1). This effect was not associated with changes in body weight or BMI, although DEXA revealed significant decreases in central measures of fat mass (Watts *et al.*, 2005). Training was also associated with enhanced insulin resistance (Bell *et al.*, 2007), as indicated by euglycaemic hyperinsulinaemic clamp technique (Figure 3.2) and improvement in diastolic function (Sharpe *et al.*, 2006; Naylor *et al.*, 2008). Taken together, these data suggest that exercise training is a powerful intervention which normalises vascular, cardiac and metabolic function in young people at high risk of future manifestations of atherosclerotic cardiovascular disease.

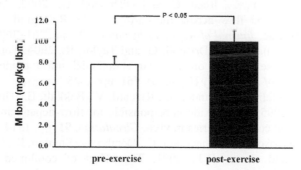

Figure 3.2. Effect of exercise training on insulin resistance assessed via euglycaemic hyperinsulinaemic clamp (14 obese adolescents). Exercise training improves, but does not normalise, insulin sensitivity in obese adolescents (Bell *et al.*, 2007).

3.7 SUMMARY

Exercise training improves vascular function and induces arterial remodelling in vivo. These effects are associated with the direct impact of episodic changes in shear stress during repeated bouts of exercise. Such direct "vascular conditioning" effects provide a plausible mechanistic explanation for some of the cardioprotective benefits of exercise. However, different types or forms of exercise, and perhaps even different intensities, are associated with different antegrade and retrograde shear stress patterns. Training benefits may therefore depend upon the nature of the shear stress stimulus involved in the exercise.

The beneficial effects of exercise training that we have demonstrated in type 2 diabetic subjects, and children and adolescents with obesity, include enhanced vascular function, cardiac diastolic function and insulin sensitivity. The effects should decrease the risk of future cardiovascular events in young people at high risk. Exercise and increases in physical activity levels are a key preventative health strategy in young people.

3.8   REFERENCES

Bell, L.M., Watts, K., Siafarikas, A., Thompson, A., Ratnam, N., Bulsara, M., Finn, J., O'Driscoll, G., Green, D.J., Jones, T.W. and Davis, E.A., 2007, Exercise alone reduces insulin resistance in obese children independently of changes in body composition. *Journal of Clinical Endocrinology and Metabolism*, **92**, pp. 4230–4235.

Green, D.J., Bilsborough, W., Naylor, L.H., Reed, C., Wright, J., O'Driscoll, G. and Walsh, J.H., 2005, Comparison of forearm blood flow responses to incremental handgrip and cycle ergometer exercise: Relative contribution of nitric oxide. *Journal of Physiology* (London), **562**, pp. 617–628.

Green, D.J., Cheetham, C., Reed, C. and O'Driscoll, G., 2002, Assessment of brachial artery blood flow across the cardiac cycle: Retrograde flows during lower limb exercise. *Journal of Applied Physiology*, **93**, pp. 361–368.

Green, D.J., Maiorana, A.J., O'Driscoll, G. and Taylor, R., 2004, Topical Review: Effects of exercise training on vascular endothelial nitric oxide function in humans. *Journal of Physiology* (London), **561**, pp. 1–25.

Joannides, R., Haefeli, W.E., Linder, L., Richard, V., Bakkali, E., Thuillez, C. and Lüscher, T.F., 1995, Nitric oxide is responsible for flow-dependent dilatation of human peripheral conduit arteries in vivo. *Circulation,* **91**, pp. 1314-1319.

Maiorana, A., O'Driscoll, G., Cheetham, C., Dembo, L., Stanton, K., Goodman, C., Taylor, R.R. and Green, D.J., 2001, The effect of combined aerobic and resistance exercise training on vascular function in type 2 diabetes. *Journal of the American College of Cardiology*, **38**, pp. 860–866.

Maiorana, A., O'Driscoll, G., Goodman, C., Taylor, R.R. and Green, D.J., 2002, Combined aerobic and resistance exercise improves glycemic control and fitness in type 2 diabetes. *Diabetes Research and Clinical Practice*, **56**, pp. 115–123.

Naghavi, M., *et al.* 2003, From vulnerable plaque to vulnerable patient: A call for new definitions and risk. *Assessment Strategies*: Part I., Circulation, **108**, pp. 1664–1672.

Naylor, L.H., Watts, K., Sharpe, J.A., Jones, T.W., Davis, E.A., Thompson, A.M., Ramsay, J.M., O'Driscoll, G. and Green, D.J., 2008, Effect of resistance exercise training on diastolic myocardial tissue velocity in obese children. *Medicine and Science in Sports and Exercise*, **40**, pp. 2027–2032.

Olshansky, S.J., Passaro, D.J., Hershow, R.C., Layden, J., Carnes, B.A., Brody, J., Hayflick, L., Butler, R.N., Allison, D.B. and Ludwig, D.S., 2005, A Potential Decline in Life Expectancy in the United States in the 21st Century. *New England Journal of Medicine*, **352**, pp. 1138–1145.

Sharpe, J.A., Naylor, L.H., Jones, T.W., Davis, E.A., O'Driscoll, G., Ramsay, J. and Green, D.J., 2006, Impact of obesity on left ventricular structure and diastolic function in children. *American Journal of Cardiology*, **98**, pp. 691–693.

Tinken, T.M., Thijssen, D.H.J., Black, M.A., Cable, N.T. and Green, D.J., 2008, Conduit artery functional adaptation is reversible and precedes structural changes to exercise training in humans. *Journal of Physiology* (London), **586**, pp. 5003–5012.

Tinken, T.M., Thijssen, D.H.J., Hopkins, N.D., Dawson, E.A., Cable, N.T. and Green D.J., 2009, Shear stress mediates vascular adaptations to exercise training in humans. *Journal of the Amecican College of Cardiology*, Submitted.

Watts, K., Beye, P., Siafarikas, A., Davis, E.A., Jones, T.W., O'Driscoll, G. and Green, D.J., 2004a, Exercise training normalises vascular dysfunction and improves central adiposity in obese adolescents. *Journal of the American College of Cardiology*, **43**, pp. 1823–1827.

Watts, K., Beye, P., Siafarikas, A., Jones, T., Davis, E. and Green, D.J., 2004b, Exercise training in obese children: Effects on vascular function and body composition. *Journal of Pediatrics*, **144**, pp. 620–625.

Watts, K., Davis, E., Jones T. and Green, D.J., 2005, Effect of exercise training in obese children and adolescents. *Sports Medicine*, **35**, pp. 1–18.

CHAPTER NUMBER 4

Fatigue Mechanisms in Children

C.A. Williams

Children's Health and Exercise Research Centre, School of Sport and Health
Sciences, University of Exeter, UK

4.1   INTRODUCTION

In adult physiological studies, muscle fatigue is a well studied phenomenon.
However, with children the study of fatigue has not attracted as much research.
This is surprising given that the ultimate consequence of fatigue i.e. the decline in
muscle performance, is found as readily in children as it is in adults. To a
physically active child this decline in muscle performance will have been regularly
experienced.

There are numerous definitions of fatigue but a commonly accepted one is
'any exercise-induced reduction in the maximal capacity to generate force or
power output' (Vollestad, 1997, p. 220). Another definition by Edwards (1983) is
the 'failure to maintain the required or expected force or power output' (p. 3).
"Edwards" (1983) model of fatigue, proposed as an inhibition of force, represented
fatigue that could reside in one or several sites of the chain of command that result
in force contraction. This chain of command which encompasses activation and
stimulation from the brain and central nervous system to the stimulation and
relaxation of the muscles itself has resulted in fatigue being divided into two
categories. Firstly, central fatigue which involves the central nervous system and
nervous pathways and secondly, peripheral fatigue that resides from the
neuromuscular junction to the muscle. One of the difficulties in quantifying the
degree of fatigue in children has been the use of invasive methodologies which
have been prevalent in adult studies (Williams and Ratel, 2009). In studies of
fatigue with children, external measures such as mechanical power output have had
to be relied upon to infer fatigue. The Wingate test (WAnT) with its fatigue index
was often used to quantify fatiguing processes during maximal intensity cycling.
Other tests of time to exhaustion, time trials or protocols using different
contraction types have also been used with some success. Instruments such as
electromyography (EMG), ^{31}P magnetic resonance spectroscopy (^{31}P-MRS) and
evoked twitch interpolated techniques have been utilised in an effort to investigate
causal factors of fatigue. In the paediatric literature accumulated results have
shown that there is a trend that children are able to resist fatigue better than adults
during exercise. These findings have typically used measurements of mechanical
force or power output profiles during sustained maximal isometric and repeated
bouts of high-intensity dynamic exercises. More recent evidence has shown that

boys can recover faster than men following submaximal isometric plantar flexion exercise (Hatzikotoulas *et al.*, 2009).

The observation of better resistance to fatigue in children may be explained by muscle characteristics which are quantitatively and qualitatively different to those of adults. These characteristics include the amounts of recruited muscle mass and the absolute work rates during exercise. Currently, it is an accepted tenet that children are equipped better for oxidative than glycolytic pathways. This metabolic profile results in children's lesser production and better clearance of muscle by-products inhibiting to contraction, as well as, a faster resynthesis of initial creatine phosphate stores necessary to the reconstitution of muscle power following exercise. The lower accumulation of muscle by-products found in children may be indicative of a reduced metabolic signal which would induce lower ratings of perceived exertions. From neuromuscular studies, some reports have indicated that children's lesser ability to activate their type II motor units would also explain a greater resistance to fatigue. The findings based on fatigue of agonist and antagonist muscles during isokinetic tests showed that higher levels of muscle co-activation with advancing muscle fatigue are similar in children and adults (Paraschos *et al.*, 2007). It is interesting to observe that during fatiguing intermittent running, motor efficiency is less disturbed in young children compared with adults. In fact, the lower decrease in running velocity in children is related to their lower decline in step rate because the shortening in step length is similar in children and adults.

4.2   METHODOLOGY TO ASSESS FATIGUE

There are a range of methodological assessments that can be used in the measurement of fatigue. These include maximal voluntary force, power output, endurance time, EMG, tetanic forces, low frequency twitch measures and twitch interpolation (Vollestad, 1997). In studies with children and adolescents the most common methods are the use of maximal voluntary force, power output, endurance time and EMG. This is largely a consequence of their ease of use, reliability and their ethical approval as compared to the twitch interpolation technique which is painful and unlikely to be well tolerated by children. The reliability of the assessment of fatigue is an important one and often overlooked. In the use of the maximal voluntary contraction method, the force generated can be reduced if the child is not motivated or has not learnt the skill to initiate a "best effort." As the ability to measure this force is crucial to the study of fatigue, more information is needed on these reliability issues. For example, the only way to truly determine if a voluntary effort is "maximal" is to supersede the contraction with an electrical tetanic stimulation. If the electrical stimulation does not evoke a force response greater than the voluntary one, then a maximal effort is judged to have occurred. In children, this is not practical and researchers are likely to have difficulty obtaining ethical approval. Other direct and reliable non invasive measures of fatigue are available. In one such study De Ste Croix found the maximal voluntary contractions of knee extensors during a fatiguing protocol to be reliable (coefficient of variation up to 5.4 %). Laboratory measures using endurance time as a basis for examining fluid ingestion and fatigue during cycling performance have been found to have a typical error of up to 7.3 % (Montfort-Steiger *et al.*, 2005).

During the measurement of mechanical power output, usually during cycle ergometry, the decline in the power output is most often investigated by measuring the temporal change in mechanical power output. The most common test is the Wingate test comprising peak power (usually within 1 or 5-s), mean power (averaged over 30-s) and total work done. Repeated sprint tests and the fatigue index, representing the decline in performance, have also been used. However, this has been criticised as being an unreliable measure (Oliver *et al.*, 2007). Therefore, its use is questioned.

The use of EMG during maximal voluntary isometric or dynamic single leg contractions or during submaximal cycling is commonly utilised. The electrical activity of superficial muscles via the amplitude and power spectrum of the signal can be assessed. The number and size of action potentials for the muscle of interest is a reflection of the amplitude. Thus changes in numbers of active fibres or activation can be detected but it is not possible to differentiate between the two. During isometric maximal contractions EMG amplitude falls progressively, which is often attributed to the gradual decline in the motor unit excitation rate. EMG recorded during submaximal repetitive or sustained contractions shows the opposite, a gradual rise. This is most probably due to muscle recruitment as previously recruited fibres fatigue and drop out only to be replaced by additional fibres which are recruited so as to maintain the force or power output. In one study by Hatzikotoulas *et al.* (2009) EMG activity of the soleus, medial gastrocnemius and tibialis anterior of prepubescent boys and men were found to increase similarly following submaximal isometric plantar and dorsal flexion. Despite the findings of similar fatigue levels in boys and men, the boys recovered faster for torque, soleus and medial gastrocnemius EMG (all normalised to the maximum achieved prior to the fatiguing exercise). Due to its ease of use and as a non invasive technique more protocols should utilise EMG.

Although muscle biopsies are often used in adult studies of fatigue it is not a viable option with children. However, exciting developments with ^{31}P-MRS could be considered as a tool for assessing the mechanisms of fatigue within the exercising muscle (Williams and Ratel, 2009).

4.3 CURRENT DEVELOPMENTS

It is likely that advances in technology will have a significant part to play in the investigations of fatigue in children. As instrumentation becomes more sophisticated and procedures become less invasive and therefore applicable to children, more valid experimentation can be established. A prime example is the use of magnetic resonance. Although expensive, magnet resonance scanning costs are decreasing and the size of the magnet bore is increasing to allow exercise to take place within the magnet. Other advancements in instrumentation include near infrared spectroscopy and thermoregulatory telemetry ingestible pills, both of which should allow measurement of oxy- and deoxyhemoglobin and temperature, as mechanisms of fatigue during exercise.

4.4   CONCLUSION

For such a common phenomenon as fatigue, it is surprising how little data there are on children's tolerance to exercise. To date the study of fatigue has largely been confined to the utilisation of external measurements of mechanical power output, supplemented by the additional measurement of EMG. However, there appears to be very little data on the force-time or power-time duration relationships. Considering the number of children engaged in exercise and sporting competitions, more needs to be known about the fatiguing effects of these activities. More paediatric studies involving the use of non-invasive instruments which are able to determine the mechanisms underlying fatigue are therefore warranted. These studies need to be both field and laboratory based.

4.5   REFERENCES

De Ste Croix, M.B.A., Armstrong, N. and Welsman, J., 2003, The reliability of an isokinetic knee muscle endurance test in young children. *Pediatric Exercise Science*, **15**, pp. 313–323.

Edwards, R.H.T., 1983, Biochemical basis of fatigue in exericse performance: catastrophe theory of muscular fatigue. In: H.G. Knuttgen, J.H. Vogel, and J.H. Poortmaas (eds.), International Series of Sports Science, **13**, pp. 3–28. Boston: Biochemistry Exercise.

Hatzikotoulas, K., Patikas, D., Bassa, E., Hadjileontiadis, L., Koutedakis, Y. and Kotzamanidis, C., 2009, Submaximal fatigue and recovery in boys and men. *International Journal of Sports Medicine*, **30**, pp. 1–6.

Montfort-Steiger, V., Williams, C.A. and Armstrong, N., 2005, The reproducibility of an endurance performance test in adolescent cyclists. *European Journal of Applied Physiology*, **94**, pp. 618–625.

Oliver, J.L., 2007, Is a fatigue index a worthwhile measure of repeated sprint ability. *Journal of Science and Medicine in Sport*, **12**, pp. 20–23.

Paraschos, I., Hassani, A., Bassa, E., Hatzikotoulas, K., Patikas, D. and Kotzamanidis, C., 2007, Fatigue differences between adults and prepubertal males. *International Journal of Sports Medicine*, **28**, pp. 958–963.

Williams, C.A. and Ratel, S., 2009, Human Muscle Fatigue. Routledge, London.

Vollestad, N.K., 1997, Measurement of human muscle fatigue. *Journal of Neuroscience Methods*, **74**, pp. 219–227.

The Ventilatory Response to Exercise in Healthy Children and Children with Respiratory Pathology

S. Matecki

Service central de physiologie clinique, INSERM ERI 25, Hôpital ADV
Montpellier, France

5.1 INTRODUCTION

Ventilatory function is the first step of the oxygen delivery chain. It is the link between ambient air (the source of oxygen) and the muscle, which is the main localization of oxygen consumption (VO_2) during exercise. Indeed, oxygen is necessary for the energetic metabolism of the muscle which synthesizes ATP from the oxidation of glucose and fatty acid, producing CO_2, which must return to ambient air via the same chain delivery. The ventilator response to exercise is necessary to adapt the ventilatory pump to the muscle metabolic rate as attested to by the stability of blood PO_2, PCO_2 and pH. The second step of the oxygen delivery chain is cardiovascular function. Both steps are tightly linked. Indeed, to face the increasing muscle metabolic rate during exercise, both must adapt homogeneously with an increase of minute volume. Minute volume is the product of a time parameter (breath frequency or heart beat per minute for steps 1 and 2, respectively) and a volume parameter (tidal volume or stroke volume for steps 1 and 2, respectively). The number of oxygen molecules transported per minute is equivalent in both steps, the only difference being the composition of what is being transported (gas or liquid for steps 1 and 2, respectively).

The cardiovascular response to exercise is difficult to measure but quite simple to interpret. Indeed, minute volume, which is the cardiac output at all ages, is closely linked to metabolic rate, both at rest and during exercise. On contrary, ventilatory function is easy to measure with a simple pneumotachograph, due to its direct interface with atmospheric air. Thus, the ventilatory response to exercise has been largely studied in adults, infants and in different pathologies. Nevertheless, interpretation of ventilatory parameter values obtained in this manner is complex. Indeed, the ventilatory response to exercise is under the control of two major pathways which both target the pontomedullary rhythm and pattern generator: a feed-back control including central and peripheral chemoreceptors, and a feed-forward control mainly including motor cortical output, mechanoreceptors and nociceptors from the muscles, tendons, airways and the lungs.

In this article, we will particularly focus on aspects of the ventilatory response to exercise that are specific to the pediatric population, as well as provide a short summary of the similarities with adults.

5.2   THE VENTILATORY RESPONSE TO EXERCISE IN CHILDREN: SIMILARITIES WITH THE ADULT MODEL

In adults as for infants, minute ventilation ($\dot{V}_E$) during exercise rises to meet the increased demand for blood oxygenation and CO_2 removal. The ventilatory response during incremental exercise to exhaustion has been the most largely evaluated in different populations. Indeed, maximal exercise testing represents a well standardized protocol allowing in at the same time evaluation of several important clinical parameters such as maximal oxygen uptake ($\dot{V}O_2max$), cardiovascular and muscular responses as well as the determination of limiting factors.

The mechanisms subserving the ventilatory response during exercise remain controversial, but in clinical practice, feedback control, through central and peripheral chemoreceptors, is considered the main mechanism responsible for the changes in $\dot{V}_E$ during maximal exercise testing. During the early course of incremental exercise to exhaustion, although both types of metabolism (aerobic and anaerobic) are solicited, the total CO_2 production, which is the main stimulus for the chemoreceptors, comes from aerobic metabolism. Indeed, the lactate produced by anaerobic metabolism is oxidized by the aerobic metabolism pathway to produce ATP. Thus, during this phase, $\dot{V}_E$ rises in proportion to power output, oxygen consumption ($\dot{V}O_2$) and carbon dioxide production ($\dot{V}CO_2$).

Then, in the normal fit adult, at approximately 50-60 % $\dot{V}O_2$ max, due to an increased solicitation of energetic metabolism to meet muscle ATP production demand, the level of lactate production by anaerobic metabolism overcomes the maximal rate of lactate oxidation by aerobic metabolism. The result of this inadequate equilibrium is a blood lactate accumulation buffered by bicarbonate, resulting in excessive CO_2 production beyond that generated by aerobic metabolism. This additional metabolic CO_2 production, triggers $\dot{V}_E$ in the same way as the CO_2 coming from aerobic metabolism. The consequence is a supplemental rise in $\dot{V}_E$ at a disproportionately greater rate than $\dot{V}O_2$ and power output, but not $\dot{V}CO_2$, which is the classical anaerobic threshold value but should be better referred to as ventilatory threshold number one (ATS/ACCP, 2003).

Subsequently, at approximately 80% of $\dot{V}O_2max$, blood lactate accumulation outstrips buffering capacity. The result is a metabolic acidosis which is a powerful ventilatory stimulus, responsible for a further sudden rise in $\dot{V}_E$ at a disproportionately greater rate than the $\dot{V}CO_2$, so called the ventilatory threshold number 2. This second ventilatory threshold is rarely described in young children, probably due to their lower glycolytic activity and thus a lower level of lactate production (Eriksson *et al.*, 1971).

In adults, the ventilatory response to maximal exercise testing allows the individual to maintain stability of blood PO_2, PCO_2 and pH, except at highest intensity level of exercise, above the second ventilatory threshold number at which point pH decreases as well as PCO_2 due to ventilation which is disproportionately high relative to $\dot{V}CO_2$. This feed-back metabolic control of ventilation is also present in infants. However, as compared to the adult, important differences in ventilatory responses to exercise exist and must be recognized in order to be able to correctly interpret maximal exercise testing in the infant.

5.3 VENTILATORY RESPONSE TO EXERCISE IN HEALTHY CHILDREN

The breathing pattern comes from the central drive output from the pontomedullary rhythm and pattern generator to the respiratory muscles. Minute ventilation is the result of a breathing pattern composed by two independent variables: Tidal volume (Vt) × Breathing frequency (f). Moreover, breathing frequency is the result of two dependent respiratory timing parameters, which are inspiratory time (Ti) and expiratory time (Te).

5.3.1 Tidal volume during maximal exercise testing

In adults, using a mouthpiece attached to a T piece and pneumotachograph, connected with a system of auditory feedback at different percentages of inspired CO_2, Rafferty and Gardner (1996) have clearly demonstrated that at rest, the Vt is under the strong control of metabolic feed-back, presumably to ensure adequate blood homeostasis. On the other hand, these authors observed that timing parameters (Ti, Te) were a non-metabolic function of breathing, probably under control of a feed-forward system including central command as well as muscle and lung reflexes, more appropriate for the behavioral The strong metabolic feed-back control of Vt seems also to be true in infants during exercise.

In this regard, several studies (Rutenfranz *et al.*, 1981; Prioux *et al.*, 1997) have observed a linear rise of Vt at maximal exercise (Vtmax) with age until 15 years for boys and 13 years for girls. The Vt max relative to body weight remains constant during childhood years. This strong metabolic feed-back control during exercise is confirmed by Mercier *et al.* (1991), who observed that lean body mass remained the anthropometric factor that accounted for the greatest percentage of variance (77%). Indeed, these authors described a scaling factor near one between body weight and Vt max, indicating a constant Vt max relative to body weight during growth. The same evolution was also observed during submaximal exercise. Thus, in clinical practice, a Vt max of around 30 ml/kg has been proposed (Prioux *et al.*, 1997) for boys and girls with an increase in post puberty, mainly due to the development of energetic metabolism under the stimulation of exercise. Thus, healthy children never demonstrate a "shallow breathing" pattern during exercise, and Vt is under the strong control of muscle mass which drives the metabolic feed back control.

5.3.2 Respiratory timing parameters during maximal exercise testing

As suggested by Raferty *et al.* (1996), respiratory timing parameters are under the main control of a feed-forward mechanism including central command as well as muscle and lung reflexes.

During exercise, a change in Ti and Te at a constant Vt has a direct impact on the work of breathing (Younes and Kivinen, 1984). Indeed, in adults a ratio of inspiratory time to total time of the respiratory cycle of 0.5 (Ti/Ttot = 0.5), represents the most economical pattern to minimize the work of breathing and maintain metabolic homeostasis. At maximal exercise, healthy children during growth also present a remarkably constant Ti/Ttot which approximates 0.5 (Mercier *et al.*, 1991). These results are in favor of an early maturity of the child's central ventilatory drive, which seems to produce the most economical breathing pattern during exercise.

However, when one examines breathing frequency, this is not always true. Indeed, at maximal exercise, breathing frequency shows a slow decrease with age, from 53 ± 7 at 11 years to 46 ± 7 breath per minute at 16 years, and a weak relationship to body dimension (Prioux *et al.*, 1997). Moreover, at submaximal exercise, Rowland and Cunningham (1997) suggest in infants the presence of a blunted breathing frequency rise at high work load compared to adults. But it is quite difficult to appreciate the efficiency of the child's breathing frequency during exercise in regard to the best economy to maintain metabolic homeostasis. This efficiency can be approached by evaluating ventilation at maximal exercise ($\dot{V}_E$ max), during growth. Although lean body mass was found to explain the greatest percentage of variance in $\dot{V}_E$ max, the allometric factor for $\dot{V}_E$ max and lean body mass were below 1 (0.79). This indicates that in contrast to Vt max per kg which is constant, $\dot{V}_E$ per kg decreases with growth (Mercier *et al.*, 1991). This ventilatory inefficiency at early stages of growth has been found by Andersen *et al.* (1974) who observed a progressive decrease with age in the ventilatory equivalents at maximal and sub maximal exercise. Thus young children hyperventilate during exercise, due to a high breathing frequency. This hyperventilation decreases with growth, and approaches adult values at around 16 years. An immaturity of feed back or feed forward mechanisms could be involved.

5.3.2.1 *Hyperventilation in children: implication of a feed back mechanism*

The feed back metabolic control of ventilation which stimulates the rhythm and pattern generator implies that $\dot{V}_E$ responds more closely to the demands for CO_2 clearance than O_2 uptake at any work rate according to the Fick equation:

$\dot{V}_{E\ BTPS} = (863 \times \dot{V}CO_{2\ STPD})/(PaCO_2 \times (1-V_D/V_t)$, where $\dot{V}CO_2$ is the CO_2 production, $PaCO_2$ is arterial CO_2 pressure and V_D is the dead space.

During growth, the ratio of $\dot{V}CO_2$ or Vt per kg of body weight as well as the V_D/V_t ratio stay constant during growth. Thus, $PaCO_2$ is the only parameter that may be implicated to explain the progressive decline of the $\dot{V}_E$ /kg of body weight ratio with growth. Indeed, Gratas-Delamarche *et al.* (1993) found that prepubertal boys have a lower CO_2 sensitivity threshold, and present a greater slope of the linear relation between minute ventilation and end-tidal PCO_2. These results supported by others (Cooper *et al.*, 1987) are in favor of a lower CO_2 set point at the central chemoreceptor level, which progressively increases with growth to reach adult values. Although this physiological observation is plausible to explain the high value of $\dot{V}_E$/kg ratio or ventilation equivalents in young infants, it fails to explain why secondary to a lower CO_2 set point, only breathing frequency is higher (i.e., a rapid but not shallow breathing pattern).

5.3.2.2 Hyperventilation in children: implication of a feed forward mechanism

The central output of the rhythm and pattern generator to respiratory muscles is also under the influence of neural stimulation from the thorax, the contracting muscles and the cortex. Indeed, the load imposed upon the respiratory muscles by the respiratory system, which is the sum of elastic loads (tissue resistance of the chest wall and the lung), and flow-resistive load (airway dimensions), via mechanoreceptors or nociceptors, stimulates the rhythm and pattern generator. The result is an optimization of the breathing pattern to minimize the work of breathing. By measuring mouth occlusion pressure Gaultier *et al.* (1981) have suggested that the central output to the respiratory muscles is high in young infants and decreases progressively with growth to reach adult values. These results may be related to a progressive decrease of the load imposed to the respiratory muscles. Indeed, with age children present a progressive decrease of airway resistance and increase of lung and thoracic compliance (Lanteri and Sly, 1993). Moreover, the absolute values of the scaling factor of these two parameters relative to height are different, indicating a different rate of change with growth. Thus the rhythm and pattern generator must constantly integrate a change in the stimulation pattern coming from the different mechanoreceptors or nociceptors of the respiratory system. This constant evolution of respiratory system mechanics in the child could maintain a certain immaturity of the rhythm and pattern generator to produce the optimized central output for the most economical breathing pattern during exercise.

Additional mechanisms other than immaturity could also be involved to explain the rapid but not shallow breathing observed in young infants during exercise. Mador (1991) has observed in adults that a previous induction of respiratory muscle fatigue, obtained after breathing against an inspiratory load, produces the same breathing pattern as high level exercise intensity. Indeed, the fatiguing contracting respiratory muscle, via the afferent signals from nociceptors, could stimulate the rhythm and pattern generator to produce in response a rapid but not shallow breathing. Using magnetic stimulation, Johnson *et al.* (1993) have observed that maximal exercise testing alone, may induce respiratory muscle fatigue. Respiratory muscle fatigue during exercise can be decreased by unloading the respiratory muscles with non invasive mechanical ventilation. Using this model, previous studies have observed during incremental exercise in the unloaded group compared to controls, a less important increase of $\dot{V}_E$, breathing fresquency and dyspnea with no difference in Vt (Babcock *et al.*, 2002; Harms *et al.*, 2000).

This respiratory sensation decrease could be an important mechanism. Indeed, a more recent study made a link between respiratory discomfort and inspiratory load compensation (Raux *et al.*, 2007). At rest, using inspiratory threshold valve, this study proposed that breathing pattern adaptation to inspiratory loading could also depend on higher cortical motor areas, and thus respiratory sensation.

The sensation of respiratory discomfort during exercise in children is poorly known, as well as the susceptibility to fatigue of their respiratory muscles. At rest, using inspiratory threshold loading, Koechlin *et al.* (2005) have suggested that respiratory muscles of prepubertal infants are more susceptible to fatigue than post pubertal infants, which have a similar respiratory muscle fatigue threshold as adults. Therefore a greater susceptibility to respiratory muscle fatigue or a higher respiratory discomfort during exercise, could also partly explain the rapid but not shallow breathing observed in young infants.

Further studies are needed to confirm this different hypothesis, but especially in young children, it is more difficult to impose an external load to the respiratory muscles during exercise for the evaluation of breathing pattern strategy. An alternative approach is the evaluation of the impact of respiratory pathology, which imposes an internal load to the respiratory muscles, on the ventilatory response to exercise.

5.4 VENTILATORY RESPONSE TO EXERCISE IN CHILDREN WITH RESPIRATORY PATHOLOGY

All respiratory pathology adds a supplementary load to the respiratory muscles and thus induces via the rhythm and pattern generator a breathing pattern adaptation to exercise. Numerous studies have evaluated the influence of external loads on control of the respiratory cycle in conscious adults. Even if external loading does not reproduce the internal load imposed by the respiratory pathology, results obtained from these studies are nonetheless useful to interpret the ventilatory response to exercise in children with respiratory pathology.

5.4.1 Breathing pattern adaptation to external ventilatory load in healthy adult

5.4.1.1 At rest

Using an external respiratory apparatus, different kinds of inspiratory and expiratory loads can be applied. A plastic tube with a narrowed caliber can easily reproduce a flow-resistive load, while a threshold valve represents more of an elastic load. Both are detected by mechanoreceptors which respond to chest wall distension or negative airway and intrathoracic pressure. Active chest wall is a less potent source of information for detection of external load than negative pressure (Younes *et al.*, 1990), and thus ventilatory responses are different in regard of the type of external or internal load applied.

Low levels of inspiratory threshold loading at rest induce in conscious humans a decrease of Ti and Ti/Ttot, while Vt/Ti, Vt and $\dot{V}_E$ increase (Eastwood *et al.*, 1994). This ventilatory response increases Te and thus the time available for inspiratory muscles to recuperate increases. Moreover, the efficiency of respiratory muscle contraction, which is the ratio of the work of breathing over the O_2

consumption of respiratory muscles, increases when they are required to contract more rapidly (Cala *et al.*, 1991). Thus ventilatory responses to external inspiratory threshold loading increase respiratory muscle endurance and the ability to generate inspiratory force.

Same types of experiments performed with low levels of inspiratory resistive loading produce a completely different ventilatory response with an increase of Ti and Ti/Ttot while Vt/Ti, f and $\dot{V}_E$ decrease. The consequence is a decreased efficiency of inspiratory muscle contraction, but also a probable decrease of sensory disturbance (i.e., dyspnea) associated with the resistive load (Im Hof *et al.*, 1986). Thus the ventilatory responses of conscious humans to an added inspiratory resistive load appear to reflect a greater concern for respiratory sensation than for energy expenditure by the respiratory muscles.

5.4.1.2 During exercise

During exercise, Ramonatxo *et al.* (1991) have observed the same ventilatory response to inspiratory resistive loading as previously observed at rest, with a greater concern for respiratory sensation than for energy expenditure. But with expiratory resistive loading these authors observed a response similar to that seen with inspiratory threshold loads applied at rest. In other words, there is a strategy consistent with an attempt to increase inspiratory muscle contraction efficiency. These last results can potentially be explained by the dynamic hyperinflation induced by the expiratory resistance, with the increase of end expiratory lung volume level being correlated to exercise intensity. The consequence is a progressive decrease of the thoracic compliance which can be considered as equivalent to an inspiratory elastic load due to the issue of intrinsic positive end expiration pressure (PEEP).

Taking these various results together we can conclude that, in the face of a ventilatory load, a balance seems to exist between the need to decrease on one hand respiratory muscle energy expenditure, and on the other hand an attempt to diminish the sensation of dyspnea. This balance depends on the type of respiratory load, and the breathing pattern. Indeed, with inspiratory resistive loading, the breathing pattern strategy does not necessarily adjust to achieve a situation in which the work of breathing is minimal, but rather toward an improvement in respiratory sensation. These considerations will help us to analyze ventilatory responses to exercise in children with respiratory pathologies.

5.4.2 Breathing pattern adaptation to internal ventilatory load in children with respiratory pathology

Two main characteristics of the ventilatory response to exercise are commonly found in children with respiratory pathology, and similar to the adult, represent a limiting factor for maximal exercise.

The first characteristic is a decrease of the ventilatory threshold number one (the so-called anaerobic threshold), due to muscular deconditioning, in relation to a decrease of daily physical activities.

The second is a decrease of ventilatory reserve due to a decrease of maximal minute ventilation, in relation to ventilatory function impairment.

These limiting factors are not always present in pathology and depend on its severity. They are easily diagnosed with a maximal exercise testing.

However, in regard to the different types of respiratory pathology, the components of the breathing strategy may also be different.

5.4.2.1 Children with cystic fibrosis

Patients with cystic fibrosis (CF) demonstrate a progressive, severe and irreversible airway obstruction. This leads to the development of hyperinflation, which increases with further lung injury, and an elevated physiological dead space associated with alveolar ventilation-perfusion mismatch. The above results in an increase of the ventilatory load and CO_2 retention during exercise, which both will stimulate the rhythm and pattern generator via a feed forward and feed back control previously presented in the first part of this article.

In children with cystic fibrosis, Keochkerian et al. (2005) have observed during incremental exercise, compared to healthy children (ages 10-14 years), a progressive decrease in Ti and Ti/Ttot with an increase of breathing pattern and a constant Vt and breathing frequency. Moreover, they observed a parallel increase of occlusion pressure ($P_{0.1}$), which can be considered to be an index of increased respiratory drive correlated to the increased respiratory muscle load imposed by the lung pathology. These results suggest that children with cystic fibrosis adopt a breathing strategy during exercise which is similar to that observed with the induction of dynamic hyperinflation by external expiratory resistive loading in healthy subjects (Ramonatxo et al., 1991). Thus, children with cystic fibrosis appear to adopt a breathing strategy, similar to adults, which is designed to increase respiratory muscle endurance and the ability to generate inspiratory force. These results are confirmed by the negative correlation found between Ti/Ttot and a parameter of gas trapping (ratio of residual volume to total lung capacity: RV/TLC), and the positive correlation found between the relative force required for each inspiration and the ratio of RV/TLC) (Keochkerian et al., 2005).

Interestingly, the same author, in another study (Keochkerian et al., 2008) of children having similar respiratory function at rest, observed the same Ti/tot and Ti evolution during exercise, associated with a decrease of Vt and an increase of breathing frequency, respiratory equivalents and end tidal CO_2 levels (PetCO$_2$), which could be linked to respiratory muscle fatigue. Therefore, cystic fibrosis children, despite the same ventilatory function at rest and identical aerobic physical aptitudes, can demonstrate different breathing strategies during exercise. However, those who developed at maximal exercise, a rapid shallow breathing with increased PetCO$_2$, seemed to show a higher decline of FEV1 after a period of three years of follow up (Javadpour et al., 2005).

Thus, in cystic fibrosis children, the evaluation of ventilatory responses to maximal exercise is a more sensitive tool for assessing the load imposed to the respiratory muscles, and this appears to be better correlated with prognosis than the respiratory function evaluation performed at rest.

5.4.2.2   Children with asthma

Asthma is characterized by reversible airflow obstruction and hyperinflation, as well as chronic inflammation of the airways. Similar to children with CF, the load imposed on the respiratory muscles will influence the rhythm and pattern generator via feed back and feed forward mechanisms. Interestingly, the breathing pattern strategy observed during exercise is quite different from the previously described pattern observed in children with CF. Indeed, Ramonatxo *et al.* (1989) reported that in children with moderate asthma, during exercise there is a constant Ti and Ti/Ttot, with a decrease of breathing frequency and ventilatory equivalents, but an increase of Vt. This breathing pattern is similar to the one observed in healthy subjects during exercise after the addition of external inspiratory resistive loads, i.e., a strategy characterized by a greater concern for respiratory sensation than for energy expenditure. The difference in breathing pattern compared to children with CF, could be in part due to a bronchodilatory effect during exercise, with a decrease in airway obstruction which serves to prevent the dynamic hyperinflation usually observed in children with CF. This would result in a lower level of elastic mechanical load imposed upon the respiratory muscles. Indeed these authors have found in children with asthma no increase of central drive to the respiratory muscles as indicated by the identical $P_{0.1}$ change during exercise, which indirectly could be interpreted as no difference between the two groups in regard to the respiratory muscle force required during exercise.

A specificity of the rhythm and pattern generator behavior or a specific pattern of stimulation of the different mechanoreceptors from the lung could also be proposed to explain the particular breathing pattern strategies in children with mild to moderate asthma during exercise.

5.4.2.3   Children with scoliosis

Scoliosis, when of sufficient severity, may alter the ventilatory function via a decrease in lung volume due to abnormal development of the thorax and alterations of alveolar growth. The result is a decrease of respiratory system compliance, with an increase of the inspiratory elastic load placed on the respiratory muscles, which will in turn influence the rhythm and pattern generator via a feed back and a feed forward mechanism. At rest, young scoliotic patients present a decrease of Ti, Ti/Ttot and Vt with an increase of Vt (Ramonatxo *et al.*, 1988). This breathing pattern strategy seems similar to the one observed in infants with lung fibrosis during exercise (Renzi *et al.*, 1982) or at rest in healthy subjects after the addition of an external inspiratory elastic load (Eastwood *et al.*, 1994).

The inspiratory elastic load imposed by scoliosis is attested to by the positive correlation observed between the force required for each inspiration and the angle of scoliosis and the negative correlation with lung volume (Ramonatxo *et al.*, 1988). Thus in young children, the ventilatory response to internal elastic loading (from scoliosis) would appear to be desgined to increase respiratory muscle endurance and the ability to generate inspiratory force, in the same manner as was observed in healthy adults after addition of external inspiratory elastic loads.

5.4.2.4   Children with chronic lung disease after premature birth

Respiratory function in preterm infants is altered by several mechanisms: a) underdevelopment of the lung and chest wall anatomy, b) ineffective surfactant synthesis and clearance of lung secretions, c) barotraumas related to prolonged mechanical ventilation, and d) toxicity of oxygen supplementation. These are risks for the development of irreversible damage to the lung parenchyma and small airways, referred to as bronchopulmonary dysplasia, which is now defined as the need for supplemental oxygen support for at least 28 days after birth. Its severity is graded according to the respiratory support required near term (Jobe and Bancalari, 2001). Approximately 1.5 % of newborns are premature (less than 30 weeks) and bronchopulmonary dysplasia develops in about 20% (Baraldi and Filiponne, 2007). Paradoxically, few studies have focused on the long-term outcome of lung function and exercise capacity in later life. Some authors have reported in infants and young adults normal pulmonary function at rest (Vrijlandt *et al.*, 2006; Gross *et al.*, 1998), while others have described obstruction of small airways and a lower level of aerobic capacity and muscular strength, possibly due at least in part to a more inactive lifestyle with muscular deconditioning (Rogers *et al.*, 2005; Kilbride *et al.*, 2003).

In a preliminary study of 19 children born prematurely (less than 32 wk) and 20 control children (mean age 9 years ± 1 for both groups), we evaluated the ventilatory response to exercise. At rest in the premature group, we observed a mild degree of small airways obstruction, and a decrease of maximal inspiratory pressure. During exercise, we did not observe any differences in regard to maximal oxygen consumption and ventilatory threshold number one. On the other hand, we observed in the premature group a rapid but not shallow breathing pattern with an increase in ventilatory equivalents and no change in tidal volume per kg of lean body mass. Moreover, the respiratory load imposed on the respiratory muscles during exercise, indirectly assessed by occlusion pressure measurements, was not different between groups during exercise. Considering the relative respiratory weakness observed in the premature group, this breathing pattern could be related to a greater susceptibility to respiratory muscles fatigue or to a higher level of dyspnea during exercise.

5.5   CONCLUSION

Multiple factors influence the ventilatory response to exercise. The breathing pattern strategy during exercise is under the double control of a feedback and a feed forward mechanism. Children's ventilatory response must, in addition to the same requirements as the adult, integrate modifications during growth of body size, compliance and resistance of respiratory system, as well as energetic metabolism, rhythm and pattern generator maturity. The main difference in breathing pattern strategy in infants compared to adults concerns the breathing frequency during exercise. Indeed, young children hyperventilate during exercise because of a higher breathing frequency with a constant tidal volume per kg of lean body mass. This ventilatory inefficiency observed in young infants decreases with growth. The precise mechanisms involved are unclear. Current research data suggest the possibility of a lower respiratory muscle fatigue threshold or a lower tolerance to respiratory effort that could induce a more rapid but not shallow breathing during exercise in young children. Immaturity of the rhythm and pattern generators, which must constantly adapt to the changes with growth of respiratory muscle load, could also explain this ventilatory inefficiency. However, data regarding breathing pattern strategy in response to a ventilatory load, as adopted by infants with respiratory pathology, are not in favor of this last hypothesis. To better understand specificities of the ventilatory response to exercise in children, additional studies are needed to evaluate changes with growth of the respiratory muscle threshold fatigue and its impact on breathing pattern strategy. Furthermore, there is a clear need for studies which assess the level of dyspnea in children during exercise, taking into account its role as an alarm mechanism for triggering adaptive changes in the breathing pattern strategy during exercise.

5.6 REFERENCES

Andersen, K.L., Seliger, V., Rutenfranz, J. and Messel, S., 1974, Physical performance capacity of children in Norway. III. Respiratory responses to graded exercise loadings--population parameters in a rural community. *European Journal of Applied Physiology and Occupational Physiology*, **33**, pp. 265–274.

ATS/ACCP, 2003, Statement on cardiopulmonary exercise testing. *American Journal of Respiratory and Critical Care Medicine*, **167**, pp. 211–277.

Babcock, M.A., Pegelow, D.F., Harms, C.A. and Dempsey, J.A., 2002, Effects of respiratory muscle unloading on exercise-induced diaphragm fatigue. *Journal of Applied Physiology*, **93**, pp. 201-206.

Baraldi, E., and Filipponc, M., 2007, Chronic lung disease after premature birth. *New England Journal of Medicine*, **357**, pp. 1946-1955.

Cala, S.J., Wilcox, P., Edyvean, J., Rynn, M. and Engel, L.A., 1991, Oxygen cost of inspiratory loading: resistive vs. elastic. *Journal of Applied Physiology*, **70**, pp. 1983-1990.

Cooper, D.M., Kaplan, M.R., Baumgarten, L., Weiler-Ravell, D., Whipp, B.J. and Wasserman, K., 1987, Coupling of ventilation and CO_2 production during exercise in children. *Pediatric Research*, **21**, pp. 568-572.

Eastwood, P.R., Hillman, D.R. and Finucane, K.E., 1994, Ventilatory responses to inspiratory threshold loading and role of muscle fatigue in task failure. *Journal of Applied Physiology*, **76**, pp. 185–195.

Eriksson, B.O., Karlsson, J. and Saltin, B., 1971, Muscle metabolites during exercise in pubertal boys. *Acta Paediatrica Scandinavica*, **217**: pp. S154–S157.

Gaultier, C., Perret, L., Boule, M., Buvry, A. and Girard, F., 1981, Occlusion pressure and breathing pattern in healthy children. *Respiratory Physiology*, **46**, pp. 71–80.

Gratas-Delamarche, A., Mercier, J., Ramonatxo, M., Dassonville, J. and Prefaut, C., 1993, Ventilatory response of prepubertal boys and adults to carbon dioxide at rest and during exercise. *European Journal of Applied Physiology and Occupational Physiology*, **66**, pp. 25–30.

Gross, S.J., Iannuzzi, D.M., Kveselis, D.A. and Anbar, R.D., 1998, Effect of preterm birth on pulmonary function at school age: a prospective controlled study. *Journal of Pediatrics*, **133**, pp. 188–192.

Harms, C.A., Wetter, T.J., St Croix, C.M., Pegelow, D.F. and Dempsey, J.A., 2000, Effects of respiratory muscle work on exercise performance. *Journal of Applied Physiology*, **89**, pp. 131–138.

Im Hof, V., West, P. and Younes, M., 1986, Steady-state response of normal subjects to inspiratory resistive load. *Journal of Applied Physiology*, **60**, pp. 1471–1481.

Javadpour, S.M., Selvadurai, H., Wilkes, D.L., Schneiderman-Walker, J. and Coates, A.L., 2005, Does carbon dioxide retention during exercise predict a more rapid decline in FEV1 in cystic fibrosis? *Archives of Disease in Childhood*, **90**, pp. 792–795.

Jobe, A.H. and Bancalari, E., 2001, Bronchopulmonary dysplasia. *American Journal of Respiratory and Critical Care Medicine*, **163**, pp. 1723–1729.

Johnson, B.D., Babcock, M.A., Suman, O.E. and Dempsey, J.A., 1993, Exercise-induced diaphragmatic fatigue in healthy humans. *Journal of Physiology*, **460**, pp. 385–405.

Keochkerian, D., Chlif, M., Delanaud, S., Gauthier, R., Maingourd, Y. and Ahmaidi, S., 2005, Timing and driving components of the breathing strategy in children with cystic fibrosis during exercise. *Pediatric Pulmonology*, **40**, pp. 449–456.

Keochkerian, D., Chlif, M., Delanaud, S., Gauthier, R., Maingourd, Y. and Ahmaidi, S. 2008, Breathing pattern adopted by children with cystic fibrosis with mild to moderate pulmonary impairment during exercise. *Respiration*, **75**, pp. 170–177.

Kilbride, H.W., Gelatt, M.C. and Sabath, R.J., 2003, Pulmonary function and exercise capacity for ELBW survivors in preadolescence: effect of neonatal chronic lung disease. *Journal of Pediatrics*, **143**, pp. 488–493.

Koechlin, C., Matecki, S., Jaber, S., Soulier, N., Prefaut, C. and Ramonatxo, M., 2005, Changes in respiratory muscle endurance during puberty. *Pediatric Pulmonology*, **40**, pp. 197–204.

Lanteri, C.J. and Sly, P.D., 1993, Changes in respiratory mechanics with age. *Journal of Applied Physiology*, **74**, pp. 369–378.

Mador, M.J., 1991, Respiratory muscle fatigue and breathing pattern. *Chest*, **100**, pp. 1430–1435.

Mercier, J., Varray, A., Ramonatxo, M., Mercier, B. and Prefaut, C., 1991, Influence of anthropometric characteristics on changes in maximal exercise ventilation and breathing pattern during growth in boys. *European Journal of Applied Physiology and Occupational Physiology*, **63**, pp. 235–241.

Prioux, J., Ramonatxo, M., Mercier, J., Granier, P., Mercier, B. and Prefaut, C., 1997, Changes in maximal exercise ventilation and breathing pattern in boys during growth: a mixed cross-sectional longitudinal study. *Acta Physiologica Scandinavica*, **161**, pp. 447–458.

Rafferty, G.F. and Gardner, W.N., 1996, Control of the respiratory cycle in conscious humans. *Journal of Applied Physiology*, **81**, pp. 1744–1753.

Ramonatxo, M., Amsalem, F.A., Mercier, J.G., Jean, R. and Prefaut, C., 1989, Ventilatory control during exercise in children with mild or moderate asthma. *Medicine and Science in Sports Exercise*, **21**, pp. 11–17.

Ramonatxo, M., Mercier, J., Cohendy, R. and Prefaut, C, 1991, Effect of resistive loads on pattern of respiratory muscle recruitment during exercise. *Journal of Applied Physiology*, **71**, pp. 1941–1948.

Ramonatxo, M., Milic-Emili, J. and Prefaut, C., 1988, Breathing pattern and load compensatory responses in young scoliotic patients. *European Respiratory Journal*, **1**, pp. 421–427.

Raux, M., Straus, C., Redolfi, S., Morelot-Panzini, C., Couturier, A., Hug, F. and Similowski, T., 2007, Electroencephalographic evidence for pre-motor cortex activation during inspiratory loading in humans. *Journal of Physiology*, **578**, pp. 569–578.

Renzi, G., Milic-Emili, J. and Grassino, A.E., 1982, The pattern of breathing in diffuse lung fibrosis. *Bulletin Europeen de Physiopatholie Respiratoire*, **18**, pp. 461–472.

Rogers, M., Fay, T.B. and Whitfield, M.F., 2005, Tomlinson J, Grunau RE: Aerobic capacity, strength, flexibility, and activity level in unimpaired extremely low birth weight (<or=800 g) survivors at 17 years of age compared with term-born control subjects. *Pediatrics*, **116**, e58–65.

Rowland, T.W. and Cunningham, L.N., 1997, Development of ventilatory responses to exercise in normal white children. A longitudinal study. *Chest*, **111**, pp. 327–332.

Rutenfranz, J., Andersen, K.L., Seliger, V., Klimmer, F., Ilmarinen, J., Ruppel, M. and Kylian, H., 1981, Exercise ventilation during the growth spurt period: comparison between two European countries. *European Journal of Pediatrics*, **136**, pp. 135–142.

Vrijlandt, E.J., Gerritsen, J., Boezen, H M., Grevink, R.G. and Duiverman, E.J., 2006, Lung function and exercise capacity in young adults born prematurely. *American Journal of Respiratory and Critical Care Medicine*, **173**, pp. 890–896.

Younes, M. and Kivinen, G., 1984, Respiratory mechanics and breathing pattern during and following maximal exercise. *Journal of Applied Physiology*, **57**, pp. 1773–1782.

Younes, M., Jung, D., Puddy, A., Giesbrecht, G. and Sanii, R., 1990, Role of the chest wall in detection of added elastic loads. *Journal of Applied Physiology*, **68**, pp. 2241–2245.

CHAPTER NUMBER 6

Daily Activities and Body Weight Stability in Children: The Unfortunate Influence of Modernity

A. Tremblay

Laval University, Canada

6.1   INTRODUCTION

The technological developments that have occurred in the last century have allowed a considerable reduction of the physical demand of daily activities. This has undoubtedly improved the efficiency and productivity of labor but for many individuals, this change in activities has removed the main source of physical stimulation contributing to optimal body functioning. In this context, leisure time physical activities have been considered as the main alternative and have been the object of a lot of advertisement for every individual. Despite this dissemination effort, adequate physical activity participation is not achieved by a majority of people, be it in children or adults, and is considered as an important determinant of overweight and obesity.

Besides the tendency of modernity to promote sedentariness, other relevant changes in daily activities have been recently observed and are worthy of consideration as determinants of childhood obesity. As discussed in this paper, the decrease in sleep duration and the increase in activities soliciting mental work also favor significant modifications of energy balance. Thus, beyond the effect of physical activity on body composition, this paper extends the discussion of this global issue to additional activities whose impact on energy balance has been unsuspected until recently.

6.2   PHYSICAL ACTIVITY AND BODY COMPOSITION

The study of the risk of excess body weight in relation to physical activities has generally been focused on their energy cost. Indeed, exercise is primarily viewed as a calorie burning agent having an impact which is essentially proportional to the amount of energy expended. Such a vision is supported by the available literature but our research experience also reveals that exercise intensity can influence energy balance. We have indeed demonstrated that calorie for calorie, vigorous physical activity exerts a more pronounced effect on post-exercise energy intake

(Imbeault *et al.*, 1997), skeletal muscle oxidative enzymes (Tremblay *et al.*, 1994), and resting metabolic rate and fat oxidation (Yoshioka *et al.*, 2001). These observations have implications regarding the opportunities of vigorous effort that are offered by sports. Indeed, sports imposing high intensity exercise are not only challenging and entertaining but they also provide the stimulus for an optimal regulation of energy balance. However, it is to be noted that the decrease in physical fitness that has been observed in children over the last decades does not spontaneously favor the adherence to activity habits which include vigorous exercise (Brunet *et al.*, 2007).

6.3   SLEEP AND BODY COMPOSITION

Sleep is an activity that contributes to the recovery of body homeostasis and it seems that this perception is valid for appetite control. Indeed, Spiegel *et al.* (2004) investigated the effects of an experimental reduction of sleep duration and found significant changes in both appetite sensations and related hormones. Specifically, they observed that sleep restriction induced an increase in the plasma concentration of the orexigenic hormone ghrelin and a decrease in plasma leptin which is known for its reducing effects on food intake. Accordingly, hunger was increased by sleep deprivation in their study.

These results prompted us to examine the relationship between sleep duration and the risk of overweight in children. A negative relationship between sleep duration and BMI was found in boys (Chaput *et al.*, 2006). Furthermore, the increased body weight characterizing the short sleeper was associated with a greater than predicted waist circumference, suggesting a preferential accumulation of fat at the abdominal level (Chaput and Tremblay, 2007). We also examined the predictability of the risk of overweight by short sleeping and other well established risk factors of excess weight in children. Interestingly, short sleep duration had a better predictive capacity of the risk of overweight compared to sedentariness and TV viewing (Chaput *et al.*, 2006).

We also used data collected in adults participating in the Quebec Family Study to better understand the metabolic correlates of body composition in short sleepers. According to the results of Spiegel *et al.* (2004), we observed that their plasma concentrations of leptin were lower than those predicted by their body fat (Chaput *et al.*, 2007). In addition, we documented a greater proneness of short and long sleepers to hypoglycemia compared to normal sleepers (Chaput *et al.*, 2007). Finally, our prospective analyses revealed that this state of mild hypoglycemia is a significant predictor of long term weight gain (Boulé *et al.*, 2008) and of the development of glucose intolerance and diabetes over time (Chaput *et al.*, 2009).

Taken together, these findings indicate that sleep is an activity that can strongly influence feeding behavior, body composition, and related metabolic and hormonal variables. In fact, we recently reported in adults that sleep duration predicted the risk of overweight to a greater extent than vigorous physical activity non-participation, high-fat diet and high-alcohol consumption (Chaput *et al.*, in press). This also lends support to the notion that obesity has a multifactorial origin.

6.4   MENTAL WORK AND FOOD INTAKE

"There is always some reluctance to admit that something we strongly wish might become a source of problems". This observation that is formulated as a maxim is not irrelevant regarding the recent evolution of our physical activity practice. Indeed, after having deployed so much effort to attenuate the physical burden of daily labor, knowledge-based work has inevitably emerged as the alternative to maintain productivity and competitiveness under free-living labor conditions. This transition has been facilitated by the availability of computers which has almost become a necessary equipment for daily transactions in every age group. In a subtle manner, computerization has also significantly increased the cognitive effort of daily activities.

Our research team has been recently interested by the impact of mental work on energy balance. Initially, this research interest was dictated by theoretical considerations pertaining to the metabolic particularities of muscle cells and neurons. Indeed, physical work solicits skeletal muscle which is metabolically equipped to oxidize both carbohydrates and fat. Conversely, mental work requires the work of neurons which essentially rely on glucose for their metabolism under normal feeding conditions. Since carbohydrate stores are limited and that lipids cannot be used as a substitute for carbohydrates when their availability is decreased, we hypothesized that mental work could have the particularity to increase spontaneous energy intake.

The first opportunity that we had to examine the possibility of a hyperphagic effect of knowledge-based work was a case study in which a scientist participated in two 60 min sessions. In one session, he had to dictate the text of a grant application whereas the second session was a control period of rest. Blood samples collected every 15-min revealed that plasma glucose and insulin instability was much greater during the mental work session (Tremblay and Therrien, 2006). In addition, hunger sensations were increased by the cognitive effort. This study was followed by additional preliminary work which showed that a 45-min session of conceptual integration and computer writing increased by 200 kcal spontaneous feeding after the session of mental work compared to a control resting session (Tremblay and Therrien, 2006).

This preliminary work was followed by a laboratory-based study in which Laval University female students were randomly submitted to two 45-min sessions (Chaput and Tremblay, 2007). The control session was a rest period whereas the experimental one consisted of a reading-computer writing session over the same time period. Interestingly, the reading-writing work had a trivial enhancing effect (3 kcal for 45 min) on energy expenditure. This strongly contrasted with the enhancing effect on ad libitum energy intake (229 kcal) that followed the session. Thus, the reading-writing session induced a short term positive energy balance of 226 kcal compared to the control condition.

In a subsequent study, we again assessed the impact of mental work on spontaneous energy intake with the additional preoccupation to assess the intensity of cognitive effort and its link with variations in plasma variables (Chaput *et al.*, 2008). In this case, we measured the impact of two 45-min sessions of mental work soliciting computer use that were compared to a control resting session. As expected, energy intake after working sessions was increased by 200 to 250 kcal after the cognitive effort compared to the rest control session. More than half of this excess energy intake was accounted by the increase in dessert consumption. Furthermore, mental work promoted an increase in cortisolemia and the instability of plasma glucose and insulin. When subjects were divided on the basis of the intensity of their cognitive effort, a significantly lower increase in energy intake, plasma cortisol and glucose instability was observed in subjects for whom cognitive effort was lower (Chaput and Tremblay, 2009; in press). Taken together, these results suggest that demanding mental work is more susceptible to induce a positive energy balance than sedentary rest.

6.5   OBESITY AND ACTIVITY: A GLOBAL CHANGE IN LIFESTYLE

The integration of messages presented above leads to the conclusion that as far as obesity is considered in relation to the evolution of daily activities, it is not only attributable to sedentariness, i.e. the insufficient participation in physical activities. These observations rather emphasize the effect of a global change in our lifestyle. Recently, Mathieu *et al.* (2009) tried to give a practical meaning to this concept by evaluating the prevalence of overweight in children at risk of obesity in relation to currently accepted guidelines for participation in physical activities, TV viewing, sleep duration, and time allocated to school homework. Interestingly, duration of sleep and school homework were independent predictors of the risk of overweight. In addition, the percentage of overweight was 26, 43, 54, and 64 in subjects deviating for 1, 2, 3, and 4 guidelines, respectively. This observation is obviously problematic since it challenges the relevance of a lifestyle that we have chosen and that contributes to our productivity and social competitiveness.

6.6   REFERENCES

Boulé, N.G., Chaput, J.P., Doucet, E., Richard, D., Després, J.P., Bouchard, C. and Tremblay, A., 2008, Glucose homeostasis predicts weight gain: prospective and clinical evidence. *Diabetes Metabolism Research and Reviews*, **24**, pp. 123–129.

Brunet, M., Chaput, J.P. and Tremblay, A., 2007, The association between low physical fitness and high BMI or waist circumference is increasing with age in children: the "Québec en Forme" project. *International Journal of Obesity*, **31**, pp. 637–643.

Chaput, J.P. and Tremblay, A. 2007, Acute effects of knowledge-based work on feeding behavior and energy intake. *Physiology Behavior*, **90**, pp. 66–72.

Chaput, J.P. and Tremblay, A., 2007, Does short sleep duration favor abdominal adiposity in children? *International Journal of Pediatric Obesity*, **2**, pp. 188–191.

Chaput, J.P. and Tremblay, A., 2009, The glucostatic theory of appetite control and the risk of obesity and diabetes. *International Journal of Obesity*, **33**, pp. 46–53.

Chaput, J.P. and Tremblay, A, Obesity and physical inactivity: the relevance to reconsider the notion of sedentariness. *Obesity Facts*, in press.

Chaput, J.P., Brunet, M. and Tremblay, A., 2006, Relationship between short sleep hours and childhood overweight/obesity: results from the "Québec en forme" Project. *International Journal of Obesity*, **30**, pp. 1080–1085.

Chaput, J.P., Després, J.P., Bouchard, C. and Tremblay, A., 2007, Short sleep duration is associated with reduced leptin levels and increased adiposity: results from the Quebec Family Study. *Obesity*, **15**, pp. 253–261.

Chaput, J.P., Després, J.P., Bouchard, C., Astrup, A. and Tremblay A., 2009, Sleep duration as a risk factor for the development of type 2 diabetes or impaired glucose tolerance: Analyses of the Quebec Family Study. *Sleep Medicine*, **10**, pp. 919–924.

Chaput, J.P., Després, J.P., Bouchard, C. and Tremblay, A., 2007, Association of sleep duration with type 2 diabetes and impaired glucose tolerance. *Diabetologia*, **50**, pp. 2298–2304.

Chaput, J.P., Drapeau, V., Poirier, P., Teasdale, N. and Tremblay, A., 2008, Glycemic instability and spontaneous energy intake: association with knowledge-based work. *Psychosomatic Medicine*, **70**, pp. 797–804.

Chaput, J.P., Leblanc, C., Pérusse, L., Després, J.P., Bouchard, C. and Tremblay, A., Risk factors for adult overweight and obesity in the Quebec Family Study: Have we been barking up the wrong tree? *Obesity*, in press.

Imbeault, P., St-Pierre, S., Alméras, N. and Tremblay, A., 1997, Acute effects of exercise on energy intake and feeding behaviour. *British Journal of Nutrition*, **77**, pp. 511–521.

Mathieu, M.E., Chaput, J.P., O'Loughlin, J., Lambert, M. and Tremblay, A., 2009, Current guidelines may protect children against overweight and abdominal obesity. *Obesity Facts*, **2**, pp. 72 (abstract).

Spiegel, K., Tasali, E., Penev, P. and Van Cauter, E., 2004, Brief communication: sleep curtailment in healthy young men is associated with decreased leptin levels, elevated ghrelin levels, and increased hunger and appetite. *Annals of Internal Medicine*, **141**, pp. 846–850.

Tremblay, A. and Therrien, F., 2006, Physical activity and body functionality: Implications for obesity prevention and treatment. *Canadian Journal of Physiology and Pharmacology*, **84**, pp. 149–156.

Tremblay, A., Simoneau, J.A. and Bouchard, C., 1994, Impact of exercise intensity on body fatness and skeletal muscle metabolism. *Metabolism*, **43**, pp. 814–818.

Yoshioka, M., Doucet, E., St-Pierre, S., Alméras, N., Richard, D., Labrie, A., Després, J.P., Bouchard, C. and Tremblay, A., 2001, Impact of high-intensity exercise on energy expenditure, lipid oxidation and body fatness. *International Journal of Obesity*, **25**, pp. 332–339.

Part II

Metabolic Syndrome and Nutrition

Metabolic Syndrome and Its Genetic Factors: A Study of Twins from Madeira and Porto Santo Islands, Portugal

P.J. Gonçalves[1], J.A. Maia[1], G.P. Beunen[2], M.A. Carvalho[3],
A.M. Brehm[3], M.J. Almeida[4], E.R. Gouveia[4], M.A. Thomis[2], and
D.L. Freitas[4]

[1]CIFI2D, and Faculty of Sport, University of Porto, Portugal; [2]Department of Biomedical Kinesiology, Faculty of Kinesiology and Rehabilitation Sciences, Katholieke Universiteit Leuven, Belgium; [3]Department of Biology, University of Madeira, Portugal; [4]Department of Physical Education and Sport, University of Madeira, Portugal

7.1   INTRODUCTION

Metabolic syndrome (MetS) is characterized by a constellation of metabolic risk factors in one individual. In children and adolescents, Ferranti et al. (2004) and Cook et al. (2003) observed a high prevalence of MetS in US. Since indicators of MetS are moderately stable from childhood and adolescence into young adulthood (Katzmarzyk et al. 2001) and that, in adults, MetS is associated with an increased risk of type 2 diabetes, cardiovascular disease, and all cause mortality, it is of great importance to study the pathogenesis of MetS. Genetic factors together with physical inactivity, unhealthy diet and overweight are the root causes of MetS (Terán-Garcia and Bouchard, 2007). As far we know, no other study has examined the role of genetic and environmental factors in the development of MetS in Portuguese children and adolescents. This study will generate more information on MetS and make it possible to devise combined intervention programs to reduce these risk factors. Hence, the purpose of the current study was to examine the genetic and environmental influences in the five indicators of the MetS.

7.2   METHODS

7.2.1 Sample, metabolic syndrome and zygosity

Data are from the 'Madeira Twin-Families Study', a cross-sectional study carried out in Autonomous Region of Madeira (ARM), Portugal. The sample comprised

207 pairs of twins, 84 MZ and 123 DZ, from 3 to 18 years of age. Pediatric MetS was defined using criteria defined by Ferranti *et al.* (2004). Blood fasting samples were taken from all participants in a private laboratory. The generated genotypes were analyzed in the Laboratory of Human Genetics of University of Madeira and subsequently the probability of monozygosity was calculated. Height was measured with a portable stadiometer (Siber-Hegner, GPM) to the nearest millimeter. Body mass was measured on a balance-beam scale accurate to 100 g (Seca Optima 760, Germany). WC was measured at the level of the narrowest point between the lower costal border and the iliac crest.

7.2.2 Statistical analyses

All analyses were performed using STATA 10 and TWINAN92 packages. Descriptive statistics were expressed as means and standard deviations (mean ± SD). Test-retest reliability for anthropometric characteristics was estimated on the basis of the intraclass correlation coefficient (R). Indicators of MetS were adjusted for age, sex and respective interactions. Genetic factors (a^2), common environment (c^2) and unique environment (e^2) were computed and models were compared by likelihood. The model retained was the more parsimonious. Statistical significance was chosen as $p < 0.05$.

7.3   RESULTS

Results of homogeneity and heterogeneity between MZ and DZ twins are given in Table 7.1. MZ twins show higher intraclass correlation coefficients than DZ twins in all indicators of MetS. Heritability (a^2) and common (c^2) and unique environments (e^2) estimates are shown in Table 7.2.

Table 7.1. Intraclass correlation (SE) in each zygosity group for anthropometric characteristics and parameters of MetS.

Indicators	MZ		DZ	
	$n^†$	M±SD	n	M±SD
WC (cm)	84	0.807±0.03	123	0.264±0.08
SBP (mm Hg)	81	0.564±0.07	122	0.308±0.08
GL (mg/dl)	84	0.559±0.08	123	0.308±0.08
HDL-cholesterol (mg/dl)	84	0.857±0.03	123	0.531±0.06
TG (mg/dl)	84	0.713±0.05	123	0.413±0.07

†Twin pairs; MZ = monozygotic; DZ = dizygotic; WC = waist circumference; SBP = systolic blood pressure; GL = fasting glucose; HDL-cholesterol = high density lipoprotein cholesterol: TG = fasting triglycerides.

Table 7.2. Estimates of heritability (a^2) common environment (c^2) and unique environment (e^2) for all indicators of MetS.

Indicators	Model[†]	a^2	c^2	e^2
WC (cm)	AE	0.80	-	0.20
SBP (mm Hg)	AE	0.59	-	0.41
GL (mg/dl)	AE	0.55	-	0.45
HDL-cholesterol (mg/dl)	ACE	0.34	0.44	0.22
TG (mg/dl)	AE	0.61	-	0.39

[†]AE = genetic additive effects and unique environment; ACE = genetic additive effects, common and unique environments; WC = waist circumference; SBP = systolic blood pressure; GL = fasting glucose; HDL-cholesterol = high density lipoprotein cholesterol: TG = fasting triglycerides.

The cluster of MetS shows heritability values (a^2) equal or higher than 0.34. Unique environment effects are comprised between 0.20 and 0.45.

7.4   DISCUSSION

Madeira genetic effects in all indicators of MetS were consistent with a previous report by Peeters *et al.* (2008) in Belgian adult twins. TG heritability in Madeira twins was higher than the estimates for HDL-cholesterol (61% versus 34%). Higher values for TG comparatively to HDL-cholesterol were also presented by Hunt *et al.* (1989). The higher TG levels together with low levels of HDL-cholesterol seemed to be associated to insulin resistance (Widén *et al.* 1992). Genetic effects for SBP in Madeira twins were higher than environmental influences. Our results parallel North-American data in adult twins (Hunt *et al.* 1989). For GL, our sample presented heritabilities of 55% of total variance. In a twin study in Caucasian children, Snider *et al.* (1999) found a similar percentage. The heritability estimate for WC was high (80%) in our sample and go beyond the known interval in the literature, namely, 25% to 40% (Terán-Garcia and Bouchard, 2007).

In the present study, environmental factors showed a low to moderate effect on the variation of the different phenotypes of MetS. This leads us to believe that different behaviors of the subjects can have a substantial influence on the total variability of phenotypes of MetS. The common environmental factor (44%) was predominant on HDL-cholesterol in comparison to unique environmental factor (22%) in Madeira sample.

The results of the current study should be interpreted in light of its strengths and weaknesses. The strengths are: (1) the sample size, more precisely, 47,7% of the total number of twins in ARM; (2) the collection of biochemical markers of MetS by expert technicians and analysis in an accredited private laboratory; (3) the determination of zygosity by the direct method. The weaknesses are: (1) the values of SM were not adjusted for biological maturation of the subjects; (2) the wide age range didn't allow performing more sophisticated analysis. In sum, this research showed that the various indicators of MS are influenced by genetic and environmental characteristics. The explained variance by genetic effects was moderate to high for WC, TG and SBP. GL was also influenced by genetic and unique environment factors, while HDL-cholesterol was predominantly influenced by environment.

7.5   ACKNOWLEDGEMENTS

The project entitled 'Genetic and environmental influences on physical activity, fitness and health: the Madeira family study' was supported by grants from the Portuguese Foundation for Science and Technology (reference POCI/DES/5683412004) and by a grant from the Centre for Macaronesian Studies. Participation of Maia, J.A. was also linked to the grant PTDC/DES/67569/2006 from the Portuguese Foundation for Science and Technology.

7.6   REFERENCES

Cook, S., Weitzman, M., Auinger, P., Nguyen, M. and Dietz, W.H., 2003, Prevalence of a metabolic syndrome phenotype in adolescents: findings from the third National Health and Nutrition Examination Survey, 1988–1994. *Archives of Pediatrics and Adolescent Medicine*, **157**, pp. 821–827.

Ferranti, D., Gauvreau, K., Ludwig, S., Neufeld, J., Newburger, W. and Rifai, N., 2004, Prevalence of the metabolic syndrome in American adolescents. Findings from the third National Health and Nutrition Examination Survey. *Circulation*, **110**, pp. 2494–2497.

Hunt, C., Hasstedt, J., Kuida, H., Stults, M., Hopkins, N. and Williams, R., 1989, Genetic heritability and common environmental components of resting and stressed blood pressures, lipids, and body mass index in Utah pedigrees and twins. *American Journal of Epidemiology*, **129**, pp. 625–638.

Katzmarzyk, T., Perusse, L., Malina, R., Bergeron, J., Depres, J. and Bouchard, C., 2001, Stability of indicators of the metabolic syndrome from childhood and adolescence to young adulthood: the Quebec Family Study. *Journal of Clinical Epidemiology*, **54**, pp. 190–195

Peeters, M., Thomis, M., Loos, R., Derom, C. Fagard, R., Vlietinck, R. and Beunen, G., 2008, Clustering of metabolic risk factors in young adults: Genes and environment. *Atherosclerosis*, **200**, pp. 168–176.

Snider, H., Boomsma, I., Doornen, J. and Neale, C., 1999, Bivariate genetic analysis of fasting insulin and glucose levels. *Genetic Epidemiology*, **16**, pp. 426–446.

Terán-Garcia, M. and Bouchard, C., 2007, Genetics of the metabolic syndrome. *Applied Physiology, Nutrition, and Metabolism*, **32**, pp. 89–114.

Widén, E., Ekstrand, A., Saloranta, C., Franssila-Kallunki, A., Eriksson, J., Schalin-Jäntti, C. and Groop, L., 1992, Insulin resistance in Type 2 (non-insulin-dependent) diabetic patients with hypertriglyceridaemia. *Diabetologia*, **35**, pp. 1140–1145.

Familiality in Metabolic Syndrome Indicators. A Study with Azorean Families

J.A. Maia, M. Campos, R. Chaves, M. Souza, D. Santos, A. Seabra, and R. Silva

CIFID and Faculty of Sport, University of Porto, Porto, Portugal

8.1 INTRODUCTION

Metabolic syndrome (MS) is an aggregate of cardiovascular risk factors. Different operational definitions of MS are available (Alberti *et al.*, 2005). Yet, there is some consensus concerning a list of five putative indicators: high systolic blood pressure, high glycemia, high triglycerides, high waist girth, and low HDL cholesterol (NCEP, 2001). Metabolic syndrome has been consistently associated with significant increases of type II diabetes, cardiovascular disease and mortality (Gami *et al.*, 2007). Its prevalence has increased over the last years not only in adults (Li and Ford, 2006), but also in children (Kim *et al.*, 2007). In addition, physical inactivity and non-healthy nutritional habits seem to play important roles in the emergence of MS. Genetic and environmental factors are the main agents in the clustering of these five metabolic risk factors at the individual and population levels. Several lines of research with families suggest that there is a moderate-to-high level of additive genetic effects (Poulsen *et al.*, 2001). It is known (Fiúza *et al.*, 2007) that the prevalence of MS of Portuguese adults is 29.4% (27.5% in males and 31.2% in females). No population information is available concerning the prevalence of MS in children, and there are no records concerning its aggregation within Portuguese families. The purposes of this study are twofold: (1) to estimate the clustering of MS in Azorean families, and (2) its genetic and environmental components.

8.2 METHODS

Azores, a transcontinental archipelago, being an autonomous region of the republic of Portugal, is located in the northwest Atlantic. It consists of nine main islands. We sampled 410 subjects belonging to 133 nuclear families from Faial (n=25 families), São Miguel (n=21 families) and Pico (n=87 families) whose age, sex and parental distribution is shown in Table 8.1

Table 8.1. Sample distribution according to age, family structure, and sex.

Age interval (years)	Father (n=114)	Mother (n=130)	Age interval (years)	Sons-daughters (n=166)	
				Males (n=91)	Females (n=75)
≤ 29	2	4	8 – 9	11	9
30 - 34	7	20	10 – 11	16	5
35 – 39	23	38	12 – 13	24	23
40 – 44	37	46	14 – 15	24	20
45 – 49	30	18	16 – 17	15	15
≥ 50	15	4	18 – 19	1	3

Physical activity was recorded with the Bouchard 3-day dairy (Bouchard *et al.*, 1983). All subjects attended their local Health Center for blood sampling after 10 hours of fasting conditions. Trained nurses took their blood, measured their blood pressure and waist girth. Triglycerides, C-HDL and Glycemia values were obtained from a single certified laboratory using standard procedures. Blood pressure measures were taken with an electronic device (Dinamap, BP 8800 model) using a standard protocol (Pickering *et al.*, 2005), and waist girth was measured in accordance with suggestions made by WHO (1989). Metabolic syndrome indicators and cut-off values were defined as suggested from different sources (NCEP, 2001; Cook *et al.*, 2003). Data analysis includes the usual descriptive statistics. Familial correlations were computed in S.A.G.E. Maximum likelihood procedures were used to estimate genetic components in each of the MS indicators using SOLAR 4.0 software.

8.3 RESULTS

Correlations among family members are presented on Table 8.2 and their patterns are low (DBP) to high (C-HDL; Glucose), suggesting familial aggregation in the different indicators of the MS. The somewhat high standard errors are due to the small sample size.

Heritability estimates are presented in Table 8.3, and all values are statistically significant, even when controlling for different covariates. Genetic factors account for low (DBP), moderate (GLU) and high (WG, SBP, C-HDL) percentage of the total variation at the population level. Even when controlled for physical activity levels, heritability estimates remain very similar to those shown in Table 8.3.

Table 8.2. Correlations±SE (intraclass for same sex members; interclass for opposite sex members) for all family members.

Relationship	WG[†]	SBP[†]	DBP[†]	C - HDL[†]	TG[†]	GLU[†]
Father-son	0.49±0.18	0.25±0.12	0.08±0.13	0.66±0.07	0.31±0.11	0.55±0.17
Mother-son	0.15±0.23	0.21±0.14	0.11±0.13	0.48±0.10	0.51±0.09	0.37±0.23
Father-daughter	0.35±0.15	0.40±0.10	0.21±0.12	0.54±0.08	0.40±0.08	0.37±0.16
Mother-daughter	0.45±0.14	0.17±0.13	-0.09±0.14	0.37±0.11	0.17±0.11	-0.21±0.19
Brother-brother	0.54±0.30	-0.22±0.64	-0.66±0.43	0.79±0.16	0.09±0.43	0.61±0.27
Sister-brother	-0.20±0.29	0.52±0.24	0.40±0.28	0.73±0.14	0.34±0.30	0.80±0.12
Sister-sister	0.45±0.23	-0.05±0.37	-0.02±0.37	0.88±0.06	-0.25±0.35	0.68±0.15
Mother-father	0.45±0.15	0.20±0.10	0.08±0.10	0.50±0.07	0.08±0.09	0.39±0.17

[†] WG= Waist Girth; SBP= Systolic Blood Pressure; DBP= Diastolic Blood Pressure; C-HDL= Cholesterol High Density Lipoprotein; TG= Triglycerides; GLU= Glucose

Table 8.3. Heritability estimates (h^2±se), p-values and significant covariates.

Phenotypes	$h^2 \pm$ se	p-value	covariates
WG	0.56 ± 0.10	<0.001	Age
SBP	0.58 ± 0.10	<0.001	Age^2; Age x Sex; Age^2 x Sex
DBP	0.19 ± 0.11	0.048	Age
C-HDL	0.77 ± 0.07	<0.001	Age; Age x Sex; Age^2 x Sex
TRI	0.65 ± 0.09	<0.001	Sex; Age x Sex; Age^2 x Sex
GLU	0.35 ± 0.11	<0.001	Age^2; Age x Sex

8.4 DISCUSSION

Metabolic syndrome indicators seem to cluster around family members. Most of the correlation coefficients are significant. These data are consistent with information provided by Lee *et al.* (2003) with the Framingham Heart Study, and the same occurred with a sample from Chinese families (Chien *et al.*, 2007). Notwithstanding the fact that heritability estimates are dependent on sample size and family structure, distribution of phenotypes, and covariate adjustments, data are consistent across studies (see Table 8.4). Genetic factors account for the variation found at the population level in MS indicators, and this importance is low to high, in accordance with the chosen phenotype.

Table 8.4. Brief summary of heritability estimates in different studies compared to the present study.

Authors (year)	Country	Sample	Origin	Phenotype					
				WG	SBP	DBP	C-HDL	TRI	GLU
Present Study	PT	410 Subjects 133 Families	Caucasian	0.56	0.58	0.19	0.77	0.65	0.35
Hsueh et al. (2000)	USA	953 Subjects 45 Families	Caucasian	0.37	0.18	0.24	0.50	0.35	0.77
Lin et al. (2005)	USA	803 Subjects 89 Families	Hispanic Caribean	0.46	0.16	0.21	0.60	0.47	0.24
Li et al. (2006)	CHN	913 Subjects 179 Families	Asiatic	0.63	0.55	0.62	0.63	0.45	0.28
Tang et al. (2006)	USA	1940 Subjects 445 Families	Caucasian	0.42	0.34	0.33	0.63	0.48	0.37

After confirming familial aggregation and significant heritability estimates in MS indicators, Phase III of Genetic Epidemiology implies genome-wide linkage studies to identify chromosomal regions that may harbor candidate genes (Arya *et al.*, 2002; Loos *et al.*, 2003), although results are not consistent in the identified chromosomal areas. This very same trend is seen in phase IV (association studies with candidate genes). In conclusion, MS indicators are found to be genetically dependent (evidence of indirect familial transmission). Their magnitude is low to high in Azorean families. Nevertheless, an important amount of inter-individual variation at family level is accounted for by environmental factors which may be linked to nutritional habits, and their body fatness, namely abdominal fat. This calls for prevention programs, aiming the family as a whole, to change their lifestyle towards a healthy one.

8.5   ACKNOWLEDGEMENTS

Portuguese Foundation for Science and Technology grant PTDC/DES/67569/2006.

8.6   REFERENCES

Alberti, K.G.M.M., Zimmet, P. and Shaw, K., 2005, The ID Epidemiology Task Force Consensus Group. The metabolic syndrome - a new worldwide definition. *Lancet,* **366**, pp. 1059–1062.

Arya, R., Blangero, J., Williams, K., Almasy, L., Dyer, T., Leach, R., O´Connell, P., Stern, M. and Duggirala, R., 2002, Factors of insulin resistance syndrome-related phenotypes are linked to genetic locations on chromosomes 6 and 7 in nondiabetic Mexican-Americans. *Diabetes,* **51**, pp. 841–847.

Bouchard, C., Tremblay, A., LeBlanc, C., Lortie, G., Savard, R. and Theriault, G., 1983, A method to access energy expenditure in children and adults. *American Journal of Clinical Nutrition,* **37**, pp. 461–467.

Chien, K., Hsu, H., Chen, W., Chen, M., Su, T. and Lee, Y., 2007, Familial aggregation of metabolic syndrome among the Chinese: Report from the Chin-Shan community family study. *Diabetes Research and Clinical Practice*, **76**, pp. 418–424.

Cook, S., Weitzman, M., Auinger, P., Nguyen, M. and Dietz, W., 2003, Prevalence of metabolic syndrome phenotype in adolescents: findings from the third National Health and Nutrition Examination Survey, 1988-1994. *Archives of Pediatrics and Adolescent Medicine*, **157**, pp. 821–827.

Fiúza, M., Martins, S. and Cortez, N., 2007, Prevalência de síndrome metabólica em Portugal - Resultados preliminares. *Revista Portuguesa de Cardiologia*, **26** (Supl II), pp. 57.

Gami, A., Witt, B., Howard, D., Erwin, P., Gami, L., Somers, V. and Montori, V., 2007, Metabolic syndrome and risk of incident cardiovascular events and death. A systematic review and meta-analysis of longitudinal studies. *Journal of the American College of Cardiology*, **49**, pp. 403–414.

Hsueh, W., Mitchell, B., Aburomia, R., Pollin, T., Sakul, H., Ehm, M., Michelsen, B., Wagner, M., Jean, P., Knowler, W., Burns, D., Bell, C. and Shuldiner, A., 2000, Diabetes in the old amish. Characterization and heritability analysis of the family diabetes study. *Diabetes Care*, **23**, pp. 595-601.

Kim, H., Park, J., Kim, H. and Kim, D., 2007, Prevalence of the metabolic syndrome in Korean adolescents aged 12-19 years from the Korean National Health and Nutrition Examination Survey 1998 and 2001. *Diabetes Research and Clinical Practice*, **75**, pp. 111–114.

Lee, K., Klein, B. and Klein, R., 2003, Familial aggregation of components of the multiple metabolic syndrome in Framingham heart and offsprings cohorts: genetics analysis workshop problem 1. *Genetics*, **4**, pp. S94–S99.

Li, C., and Ford, E., 2006, Definition of metabolic syndrome: what's new and what predicts risk? *Metabolic Syndrome and Related Disorders*, **4**, pp. 237–251.

Lin, H., Boden-Albala, B., Juo, S. and Park, N., 2005, Heritabilities of the Metabolic Syndrome and its components in the Northern Manhattan Family Study. *Diabetologia*, **48**, pp. 2006–2012.

Loos, R., Katzmarzyk, P., Rao, D., Rice, T., Leon, A., Skinner, J., Wilmore, J., Rankinen, T. and Bouchard, C., 2003, Genome-wide linkage scan for the metabolic syndrome in the HERITAGE Family Study. *The Journal of Clinical Endocrinology and Metabolism*, **88**, pp. 5935–5943.

NCEP, 2001, Executive Summary of the third Report of the national cholesterol education program (NCEP) expert panel on detection, evaluation, and treatment of high blood cholesterol in adults (adults treatment panel III). *Journal of the American Medical Association*, **285**, pp. 2486–2497.

Pickering, T., Hall, J., Appel, L., Falkner, B., Graves, J., Hill, M., Jones, D., Kurtz, T., Sheps, S. and Roccella, E., 2005, Recommendations for Blood Pressure Measurement in Humans and experimental Animals. Part 1: Blood Pressure Measurement in Humans. A Statement for Professionals from the Subcommittee of Professional and Public Education of the American Heart Association Council on High Blood Pressure Research. *Hypertension*, **45**, pp. 142–161.

Poulsen, P., Vaag, A., Kyvik, K. and Beck-Nielsen, H., 2001, Genetic versus environmental aetiology of the metabolic syndrome among male and female twins. *Diabetologia*, **44**, pp. 537–543.

Tang. W., Hong, H., Province, M., Rich, S., Hopkins, P., Arnett, D., Pankow, J., Miller, M. and Eckfeldt, J., 2006, Familial clustering for features of the metabolic syndrome. The National heart, lung, and blood institute (NLHBI) family heart study. *Diabetes Care*, **29**, pp. 631-636

WHO, 1989, Measuring obesity: classification and distribution of anthropometric data. *Copenhagen, WHO.*

CHAPTER NUMBER 9

Impact of the Built Environment on Metabolic Syndrome and Other Physiological Variables

D.R. Dengel[1], M.O. Hearst[2], J.H. Harmon[1], A. Forsyth[3], and L.A. Lytle[2]

[1]School of Kinesiology, University of Minnesota, Minneapolis, MN, USA; [2]Division of Epidemiology and Community Health, School of Public Health, University of Minnesota, Minneapolis, MN, USA; [3]Department of City and Regional Planning, Cornell University, Ithaca, NY, USA

9.1   INTRODUCTION

The built environment consists of both the micro-environment (i.e., neighborhood and street-level characteristics) and the macro-environment (i.e., level of urbanization, land-use patterns, etc.) (Swinburn et al., 1999). Not only can the built environment shape opportunities for physical activity, but it can also play a role in shaping our food intake (Humpel et al., 2002). To date, little is known about the role of the built environment on the metabolic syndrome (MetS) or other metabolic and cardiovascular diseases. Recently, we (Dengel et al., 2009) examined the relationship between the built environmental and biological markers of the MetS. This monograph will summarize and discuss the results of that study.

9.2   MATERIALS AND METHODS

We examined adolescents (ages 10-16 at baseline), who were enrolled in a 3-year longitudinal etiologic study aimed at understanding the social and environmental influences on unhealthy weight gain in adolescences. One hundred eighty-eight participants in this longitudinal study agreed to have a fasting blood sample drawn in addition to the other measures being done as part of the longitudinal study. A MetS cluster score was derived for each participant by calculating the sum of the sample-specific z-scores from percent body fat, fasting glucose, high density lipoprotein cholesterol (HDL)(negative), triglyceride, and systolic blood pressure (BP) (Kelly et al.; 2008; Dengel et al., 2009).

Geographic Information Systems (GIS) technology was used to calculate the distance to and density of pedestrian infrastructure features (e.g., transit stops), population density, land-use mix (e.g., percent land used for commercial business), street pattern (e.g., median block size), restaurants, food stores and sources of physical activity (e.g., parks) from a participant's house.

Spearman correlations were used to determine relationships between features of the built environment and the MetS cluster score and other biomarkers. Statistically significant correlations (p<0.05) were individually used in multivariate linear regression, controlling for pubertal status, age and sex.

9.3   RESULTS

The Table 9.1 below describes the characteristics of the overall study sample and the sample stratified by sex. The sample was comprised of 97 females and 91 males with average age of 15.4 yrs. The average body mass index (BMI) for the total sample was 21.6 kg/m^2 and percent body fat was 20.2%. As expected, females were further along the developmental scale, were shorter and weighed less than the males. Females also had a significantly higher percent body fat, total cholesterol, HDL, low density lipoprotein cholesterol (LDL), fasting plasma insulin and MetS cluster score than their male counterparts. Only systolic BP was lower in females than males.

Table 9.1. Characteristics of the overall study sample and the sample stratified by sex

Variable	Total (n=188)		Males (n=91)		Females (n=97)		P
	Mean	S.E.	Mean	S.E.	Mean	S.E.	
Age (yrs)	15.4	1.67	15.6	1.57	15.3	1.75	0.31
Puberty	15.2	3.29	13.6	2.95	16.7	2.87	<0.01
Height (cm)	168.2	0.71	172.9	1.07	163.7	0.68	<0.01
Weight (kg)	61.6	1.06	65.1	1.71	58.3	1.19	<0.01
BMI (kg/m^2)	21.6	3.83	21.5	3.87	21.67	3.80	0.79
Percent Body Fat (%)	20.2	9.65	13.8	7.53	26.1	7.33	<0.01
Diastolic BP (mmHg)	54.4	0.54	53.9	0.69	54.8	0.82	0.40
Systolic BP (mmHg)	115.0	9.21	117.3	9.53	112.9	8.41	<0.01
Triglycerides (mmol/L)	0.89	0.40	0.84	0.34	0.94	0.43	0.06
Total Cholesterol mmol/L)	3.86	0.06	3.64	0.07	4.06	0.08	<0.01
HDL (mmol/L)	1.27	0.29	1.20	0.31	1.33	0.27	<0.01
LDL (mmol/L)	2.18	0.04	2.00	0.06	2.30	0.07	0.01
Insulin (pmol/L)	60.1	37.8	51.8	30.8	67.9	42.1	<0.01
Glucose (mmol/L)	4.48	0.02	4.52	0.03	4.43	0.04	0.08
MetS cluster score	-0.45	3.22	-1.40	3.13	0.44	3.07	<0.01

Of the twenty-six environmental features, only the distance to convenience/gas stations was significantly (rho = -0.1634, p=0.03) related to the MetS cluster score. There was a trend (rho = -0.1320, p=0.07) for a negative association between the MetS cluster score and the percent land use dedicated to parks. Percent body fat was inversely related to the distance to fast food (rho=-

0.1447, p=0.05), but positively related to the density of small (rho=0.1699, p=0.02) and large (rho=0.2305, p=0.002) grocery stores within a 1600 m network. In addition, HDL was positively related to the distance to convenience stores (rho=0.1562, p=0.003) and a positive trend (rho=0.1233, p=0.008) was seen between HDL and the proportion of vacant land. Systolic BP pressure was significantly and inversely related to density of transit (rho=0.1861 p=0.001) and there was a negative trend (rho=-0.1349, p=0.07) seen between systolic BP and the density of large grocery stores. Multivariate linear regression revealed a statistically significant negative association between the distance to convenience/gas stations and the MetS cluster score after controlling for puberty, age and sex. We also ran multivariate linear regression on the statistically significant components of MetS and the built environment. After controlling for puberty, age and sex, we found no statistically significant relationships between the twenty-six environmental features and percent body fat or HDL. Systolic BP remained statistically significant with the density of transit (β= -22.53, SE=8.95, p=0.01) after adjustment.

9.4 DISCUSSION

The purpose of this study was to examine how the built environment impacts biological markers of MetS and if any association differs by gender. Even though the built environment and biological markers are quite distal in the causal pathway of disease, we did observe significant relationships between the distance to convenience stores and the MetS cluster score even after adjusting for pubertal status, age and gender. Although others have attempted to examine the effect of the built environment on health (de Vries *et al.*, 2003; Maas *et al.*, 2006) to our knowledge this is the first study to utilize biological markers as an indicator of health or disease.

To date, most studies examining the built environment have focused on the relationship between the distance to food outlets (i.e., driving distance or driving times) and the level of obesity (Frank *et al.*, 2007; Nielsen and Hansen, 2007). These studies have produced conflicting results at best with some studies showing a relationship between obesity levels and distance to food outlets (Frank *et al.*, 2004; Lopez-Zetina *et al.*, 2006) while others have shown no relationship (Liu *et al.*, 2002; Kelly-Schwartz *et al.*, 2004; Burdette and Whitaker, 2004; Ewing *et al.*, 2006). Our population was largely between the ages of 10 and 16 years; and few participants were able to drive independently. In the present study, we did observe a significant relationship between the distance to convenience stores and the MetS cluster score after adjusting for pubertal status, age and sex. As the distance to convenience stores increased, the MetS cluster score decreased, suggesting that the greater distance an adolescent is from a convenience store the lower the development of the MetS. It is quite possible in the present study that greater distances from convenience stores may have prevented participants from walking to or riding their bicycle to convenience stores to purchase a "snack" or beverage.

We also observed a trend for a relationship between the percent land use dedicated to parks and the MetS cluster score. Although not statistically significant the trend for significance was in the right direction and would suggest that greater access to parks and lower density of retail food outlets lowers the risk of developing the MetS. These results are in agreement with those reported by Nielsen and Hansen (Nielsen and Hansen, 2007) who reported that Danish individuals (age 18-25 yrs) who had access to green areas were less likely to be overweight/obese. Among adolescent girls from five cities in the U.S., Cohen *et al.* (2006) found that proximity to parks was associated with increased moderate and vigorous physical activity (Cohen *et al.*, 2006). Similarly, Jago *et al.* (2006) reported that access to parks was associated with physical activity levels of male adolescents. Taken together these data would suggest access to public parks and recreation areas may result in a residential environment that encourages physical activity. The result of this encouragement in physical activity may result in fewer individuals in that built environment being overweight or obese as both obesity and physical inactivity are thought to be driving factors in the development of the MetS (Park *et al.*, 2003).

There are some limitations to this study. The significant associations between the MetS cluster score, systolic BP and the built environment may not reflect actual behavior, but may be due to other factors, such as the quality of home or school food environment, or socioeconomic variations. Another limitation is that although GIS data can assess the nutrition and physical activity environment, it does not account for consumer behavior or quality of facilities or neighborhood features, such as sidewalk conditions (Forsyth, Lytle, in review). Continued refinement of GIS methodological obstacles and theory is needed to continue to advance research in this area. Finally, in the present study we used percent fat instead of BMI percentile in the actual definition of the MetS due to the fact that BMI percentile is a less sensitive indicator of fatness in children (Reilly *et al.*, 2000). We replaced percent fat with BMI percentile in our MetS cluster score and the relationship between the MetS cluster score and the distance to convenience stores remained significant (rho=-0.1717, p=0.02), suggesting that the MetS cluster score is robust.

9.5   CONCLUSION

Although this study examines the most distal associations between the built environment and biomarkers, with no attention to mediating factors, our results suggest a role for the built environment in the development of the MetS in adolescents. Additional research on biological and physiological components and the built environment with larger and more generalizable samples are needed to determine the role of the built environment on disease incidence and progression. In addition, further investigative work is needed to understand the differential relationship observed by gender.

It is important to point out that the results of this study may only be relevant to adolescents living in the United States. European cities are older and typically more compact than cities in the United States making it easier for adolescents to walk to convenience stores and other sources of food and beverage. This fact may alter some of the relationships observed in the present study. In addition, European cites often have a more developed public transit system, which again would provide adolescents with a much different built environment than what is typical in the United States.

There is one message that can be applied from this study to both European and United States cities and their youth and that is: the built environment has an effect on the overall health of our youth and most likely everyone living in that built environment. Although having convenience stores close to population centers may be important for shopping it also presents opportunities for our adolescents to engage in "unhealthy" eating habits. One way to have both access to stores and healthy adolescents may involve education such as teaching adolescents about healthy choices for beverages and snacks. In addition, the products carried by convenience stores and stores in general may also be of importance. Encouraging convenience stores to stock fruits and vegetables instead of calorically dense beverages and foods may be another way to positively shape our built environment. Finally, access to parks and free space is also important for overall health. Urban planners need to build into our cities and rural settings open space for parks and recreation. Ultimately, we have the ability to shape the environment we live in. How we choose to build our environment may actually impact the health of not only our youth, but of everyone living in that environment.

9.6 REFERENCES

Burdette, H.I., and Whitaker, R.C., 2004, Neighborhood playgrounds, fast food restaurants, and crime: relationships to overweight in low-income preschool children. *Preventive Medicine*, **38**, pp. 57–63.

Cohen, D.A., Ashwood, J.S., Scott, M.M., Overton, A., Evenson, K.R., Staten, L.K., Porter, D., McKenzic, T.L. and Catellier, D., 2006, Public parks and physical activity among adolescent girls. *Pediatrics*, **118**, pp. e1381–e1389.

Dengel, D.R., Hearst, M.O., Harmon, J.H., Forsyth, A. and Lytle, L.A., 2009, Does the built environment relate to the metabolic syndrome in adolescents? *Health and Place*, **15**, pp. 946–951.

de Vries, S., Verheij, R.A., Groenewegen, P.P. and Spreeuwenberg, P., 2003, Natural environments - health environments? An exploratory analysis of the relationship between greenspace and health. *Environment and Planning*, **35**, pp. 1717–1731.

Ewing, R., Brownson, R.C. and Berrigan, D., 2006, Relationship between urban sprawl and weight of United States youth. *American Journal of Preventive Medicine*, **31**, pp. 464–474.

Frank, L.D., Saelens, B.E., Powell, K.E. and Chapman, J.E., 2007, Stepping towards causation: Do built environments or neighborhood and travel preferences explain physical activity, driving, and obesity. *Social Science and Medicine*, **65**, pp. 1898–1914.

Frank, L.D., Andresen, M.A. and Schmid, T.L., 2004, Obesity relationships with community design, physical activity, and time spent in cars. *American Journal of Preventive Medicine*, **27**, pp. 87–96.

Forsyth, A. and Lytle, L., The neighborhood nutrition environment: assessing food sources using GIS. *Health and Place*, (under review).

Humpel, N., Owen, N. and Leslie, E., 2002, Environmental factors associated with adults' participation in physical activity—a review. *American Journal of Preventive Medicine,* **22**, pp. 188–199.

Jago, R., Baranowski, T. and Harris, M., 2006, Relationships between GIS Environmental features and adolescent male physical activity: GIS coding differences. *Journal of Physical Activity and Health*, **3**, pp. 230–242.

Kelly, A.S., Kaufman, C.L., Steniberger, J. and Dengel, D.R., 2008, Body mass index and fasting insulin explain the association between the metabolic syndrome and measures of cardiovascular risk in overweight children. *Diabetes,* **57** Supplement 1, A490.

Kelly-Schwartz, A.C., Stockard, J., Doyle, S. and Schlossberg, M., 2004, Is sprawl unhealthy? A multilevel analysis of the relationship of metropolitan sprawl to the health of individuals. *Journal of Planning Education and Research*, **24**, pp. 184–196.

Liu ,G., Cunningham, C., Downs, S., Marrero, D. and Fineberg, N., 2002, A spatial analysis of obesogenic environments for children. *Proceedings of AMIA Symposium*, pp. 459–463.

Lopez-Zetina, J., Lee, H. and Friis, R., 2006, The link between obesity and the built environment. Evidence from an ecological analysis of obesity and vehicle miles of travel in California. *Health and Place*, **12**, pp. 656–664.

Maas, J., Verheij, R.A., Groenewegen, P.P., de Vries, S. and Spreeuwenberg, P., 2006, Green space, urbanity, and health: how strong is the relation? *Journal of Epidemiology and Community Health*, **60**, pp. 587–592.

Nielsen, T.S. and Hansen, B.B., 2007, Do green areas affect health? Results from a Danish survey on the use of green areas and health indicators. *Health and Place*, **12**, pp. 839–850.

Park, Y.W., Zhu, S., Palaniappan, L., Heshka, S., Carnethon, M.R. and Heymsfield, S.B., 2003, The MetS: prevalence and associated risk factor findings in the US population from the Third National Health and Nutrition Examination Survey, 1988-1994. *Archives of Internal Medicine*, **163**, pp. 427–436.

Reilly, J.J., Dorosty, A.R. and Emmett, P.M., 2000, Identification of the obese child: adequacy of the body mass index for the clinical practice and epidemiology. *International Journal of Obesity and Related Metabolic Disorders*, **24**, pp. 1623–1627.

Swinburn, B., Egger, G. and Raza, F., 1999, Dissecting obesogenic environments: the development and application of a framework for identifying and prioritizing environmental interventions for obesity. *Preventive Medicine*, **29**, pp.563–570.

Lipoprotein(a) in Healthy Welsh Adolescents

N.E. Thomas[1], B. Davies[2], and J.S. Baker[3]

[1]Swansea University, UK; [2]University of Glamorgan, UK; [3]University of the West of Scotland, UK

10.1 INTRODUCTION

Lipoprotein(a) (Lp(a)) is a distinctive cholesterol-rich plasma lipoprotein that has a lipid composition similar to that of low-density lipoprotein (LDL). It is formed by the association of apolipoprotein(a) with apolipoprotein B 100, and considered a better marker of CVD than conventional lipids (Agoston-Coldea et al., 2008). Of the emerging CVD risk factors, Lp(a) seems to have the strongest hereditary link, and, according to Boerwinkle et al. (1992), approximately 90% of an individual's Lp(a) level can be attributed to inherited genotype.

Research evidence shows that Lp(a) levels are not normally distributed but are skewed towards low concentrations of less than 10 mg·dL^{-1} (Kronenberg et al., 1996). Although it is considered a cardiovascular risk factor; only twenty percent of Caucasians are thought to have Lp(a) concentrations greater than 30 mg·dL^{-1}, the commonly accepted cut-off point for CVD risk in both children and adults (Kronenberg et al., 1996). It is the combined elevated levels of Lp(a) and LDL-C, and Lp(a) and fibrinogen (Fg), that are believed to have the greatest detrimental effect on cardiovascular health (Cantin et al., 2002; Thomas et al., 2005).

The aim of this study was to examine established and emerging CVD risk factors in a cohort of apparently healthy adolescents. We examined the Lp(a) concentrations in schoolchildren aged 12-13 years, and the number of schoolchildren exhibiting values in excess of 30 mg·dL^{-1}. We also identified the number of participants who had combined elevated levels of Lp(a) and LDL-C, or Lp(a) and Fg.

10.2 METHODS

A cohort of 100 boys and 108 girls; aged 12.9, SD 0.3 years participated in this study. Letters of information and consent forms were distributed to the parents of all participants. Data on personal health history and familial CVD history were collected. All participants were assured of anonymity and informed that they were free to withdraw from the project at any time. The study's protocol was approved by the University's Ethics Committee.

Barefoot stature was measured to the nearest 0.001 metre using a portable stadiometer (Holtain Ltd, Pembrokeshire, UK). Body mass was recorded to the nearest 0.1 kg using a Phillips electronic scale (HP 5320), calibrated against a balanced beam scale. Blood samples were collected between 9am and 10.30am, and following an overnight fast. To control for plasma volume shifts, venous blood was sampled after the participants had assumed a seated position for at least 30 minutes (Pronk, 1993). LDL-C concentration was calculated by the Friedewald formula. Fibrinogen concentration was determined according to the method of Clauss and using the ACL Futura analyzer (Instrumentation Laboratory Company, Lexington, MA). Lp(a) concentration was measured by an immunoturbidimetric method using the Cobas Mira analyser (Roche Diagnostics, Basel, Switzerland). The laboratory analytical variance for the measurement of Lp(a) and Fg were 6% and 1.6%, respectively.

All data were analyzed using Minitab, with $P \leq 0.05$ considered significant. The Student parametric t-test was used to compare boys and girls' Lp(a), Fg, and LDL-C concentrations. Because the distribution of Lp(a) concentrations was non-continuous and highly skewed, a non-parametric Mann-Whitney U-test was used to compare gender difference.

10.3   RESULTS

No significant gender differences were identified for any of the measured variables (Table 10.1). Twenty six percent of the schoolchildren exceeded the published criterion threshold (30 mg·dL^{-1}) for Lp(a) (Table 10.2). Of those identified as having elevated levels of Lp(a), 60% reported CVD in a close family member. Three schoolchildren had combined elevated Lp(a) and LDL-C; 31 had combined elevated Lp(a) and Fg (Table 10.2).

Table 10.1. Selected characteristics and gender comparison of schoolchildren.

Variable	Boys $n = 100$ Mean (SD)	Girls $n = 108$ Mean (SD)	P value
ST (m)	1.54 (0.08)	1.55 (0.02)	
BM (kg)	50.8 (14.1)	51.8 (11.1)	
[1]Lp(a) (mg/dL)	26.9 (32)	28.5 (37.1)	0.597
LDL-C (mmol/L)	2.67 (0.70)	2.61 (0.55)	0.453
Fg (mg/dL)	402.5 (79)	389.3 (77)	0.250

ST: stature; BM: body mass; Lp(a): lipoprotein(a); LDL-C: low-density lipoprotein cholesterol; Fg: fibrinogen.[1]Values are in geometric means.

Table 10.2. Number of schoolchildren who exceeded published criterion thresholds.

Variable	Boys n = 100	Girls n = 108
Lp(a)	26	29
LDL-C	8	3
Fg	49	47
Lp(a) and LDL-C	2	1
Lp(a) and Fg	15	16

LDL-C: low-density lipoprotein cholesterol; Fg: fibrinogen; Lp(a): lipoprotein(a)

10.4   CONCLUSION

Atherosclerosis begins in childhood and progresses to CVD in adults (Groner *et al.*, 2006). Many studies have shown that elevated levels of Lp(a) are associated with atherosclerotic disease, however, it is not known whether Lp(a) elevation can be regarded as an additional risk factor in children and adolescents. The lack of consistent methodologies and reference values indicates that we are hitherto unable to establish 'normal' or 'at risk' Lp(a) levels specific to the younger population. For this reason, a cut-off point that is frequently used in young people is the value associated with adults, namely, ≥ 30 mg·dL^{-1}.

In this study, the distribution of Lp(a) levels was skewed towards the lower end, non-continuous, and over a broad range; this would explain the large standard deviation values reported. There was no significant difference between boys and girls, but 26% (*n* = 55) of the schoolchildren exceeded the published cut-off point for Lp(a). Of those schoolchildren identified as having elevated levels of Lp(a), 60% reported CVD in a close family member. Some clinicians challenge the need to measure Lp(a) as part of CVD risk assessment, particularly in the younger population, however, it is possible that Lp(a) is a risk factor worth screening for when considering the population's risk of CVD.

Elevated levels of both Lp(a) and LDL-C are considered to have the greatest detrimental influence on health status (Sveger *et al.*, 2000). In our cohort, two boys and one girl demonstrated this combination. This was similar to the value reported by Sveger and colleagues (2000) who found combined elevated levels of Lp(a) and LDL-C in 1.7% of children aged 10 to 11 years with a family history of CHD. The combination of Lp(a) and Fg was more common in our group of schoolchildren, with 15% exhibiting this unfavourable condition.

In summary, the results of this study suggest that the early identification of individuals at increased CVD risk might be worthwhile. Although lifestyle interventions, including the modification of physical activity and eating habits, are not thought to have a significant effect on Lp(a) levels, they are known to affect LDL–C and Fg. If interventions are implemented sufficiently early in life, this might reduce the potential cardiovascular risk of elevated Lp(a) which, separately, is less amenable to lifestyle changes.

10.5 REFERENCES

Agoston-Coldea, L., Mocan, T., Gatfossé, M. and Dumitrascu, D.L., 2008, The correlation of apolipoprotein B, apolipoprotein B/apolipoprotein A-I ratio and lipoprotein(a) with myocardial infarction. *Central European Journal of Medicine,* 3, pp. 381–527.

Boerwinkle, E., Leffert, C.C., Jingping, L., Lackner, C., Chiesa, G. and Hobbs, H.H., 1992, Lipoprotein(a) gene accounts for greater than 90% of the variation in plasma Lipoprotein(a) concentration. *Journal of Clinical Investigation,* 90, pp. 52–60.

Cantin, B., Després, J.P., Lamarche, B., Moorjani, S., Lupien, P.J., Bogaty, P., Bergeron, J. and Dagenais, G.R., 2002, Association of fibrinogen and lipoprotein(a) as a coronary heart disease risk factor in men (The Quebec Cardiovascular Study). *American Journal of Cardiology,* 89, pp. 662–666.

Groner, J.A., Joshi, M. and Bauer, J.A., 2006, Pediatric precursors of adult cardiovascular disease: noninvasive assessment of early vascular changes in children and adolescents *Pediatrics,* 118, pp. 1683–1691.

Kronenberg, F., Steinmetz, A., Kostner, G.M. and Dieplinger, H., 1996, Lipoprotein(a) in health and disease. *Critical Reviews in Clinical Laboratory Sciences,* 33, pp. 495–543.

Pronk, N.P., 1993, Short term effects of exercise on plasma lipids and lipoproteins in humans. *Sports Medicine,* 16, pp. 431–448.

Sveger, T., Flodmark, C.E., Nordborg K., Nilsson-Ehle, P. and Borgfors, N., 2000, Hereditary dyslipidaemias and combined risk factors in children with a family history of premature coronary artery disease. *Archives of Disease in Childhood,* 82, pp. 292–296.

Thomas, N.E., Cooper, S.M., Williams, S., Baker, J.S. and Davies, B., 2005, Coronary heart disease risk factors in young people of differing socio-economic status. *European Physical Education Review,* 11, pp. 171–187.

Immediate Effects of Exercise on Energy Intake in Normal Weight and Overweight Pre-Pubertal Children

D. Nemet[1], R. Arieli[1], Y. Meckel[2], and A. Eliakim[1]

[1]Child Health & Sports Center, Pediatric Department, Meir General Hospital, Kfar-Saba, Sackler School of Medicine, Tel-Aviv University, Israel; [2] Zinman College of Physical Education, Wingate Institute, Netanya, Israel

11.1 INTRODUCTION

Activity, or inactivity, and diet are crucial elements of life-style. Their interrelations have powerful effects on health and well-being in both adults and children. Although the mechanisms responsible for the increasing prevalence of childhood obesity are not completely understood, there is no doubt that life-style changes associated with increased energy intake and decreased energy expenditure probably play a major role (Dietz, 2004).

Animal and human adult studies suggested that appetite is suppressed and energy intake is reduced immediately after strenuous exercise. In addition, exercise-induces changes in counter-regulatory hormones (e.g. epinephrine, growth hormone) and free fatty acids resulting in increased carbohydrate and decreased fat intake immediately following exercise (Verger *et al.*, 1992). The aim of this study was to examine the immediate effect of different types of popular exercise (aerobic, resistance and swimming) on energy intake and macronutrient preferences in pre and early pubertal, normal weight and obese children. We hypothesized that following exercise the total energy intake will be reduced, and that exercise will lead to a relative increase in carbohydrate consumption. We further speculated that these changes will be more significant following aerobic exercise and swimming.

11.2 METHODS

11.2.1 Subjects

Twenty two healthy normal weight (ages 6.2-10.9 years; 5 males; 17 females) and 22 overweight and obese (ages 6.5-11 years; 7 males; 15 females) pre and early-pubertal children participated in the study.

11.2.2 Anthropometric measurements

Standard, calibrated scales and stadiometers were used to determine height, weight, and BMI (kg/m^2) at the first visit to the center. BMI-for-age percentiles were calculated and Tanner staging by breast development for females and pubic hair for males was assessed by a pediatric endocrinologist.

11.2.3 Study procedure

Children were asked to refrain from exercise each morning before the study. During the control visit (no exercise) the children watched a video movie for 45 minutes and then ate the buffet lunch. In the other three visits the participants performed three different types of typical training sessions (outdoor aerobic, indoor resistance and a swimming session). The training sessions were performed in groups of 10-12 children at a time, in random order, and lasted 45 minutes. Lunch was served within 30-45 minutes after the end of the training session.

11.2.4 Buffet lunch and nutritional assessment

A similar buffet lunch was served to the normal weight and to the overweight children after each different session (the same buffet for both groups after aerobic exercise etc.). Each participant received a numbered tray, and was told to keep that tray throughout lunch. All the foods were served to dishes that were kept on the individual tray, and the participants were instructed to leave all leftovers on the tray at the end of lunch. Meals were pre-portioned and food items were weighed to the nearest gram by the nutritionist before eating and the leftovers were weighed at the end of lunch. Any additional foods were also weighed and marked separately (e.g. second serving of a specific food or the number of drinks). Photo pictures of the trays were taken after serving and before eating, and again at the end of lunch. Food and macronutrient intake were analyzed using the Israeli Ministry of Health tables.

11.2.5 Statistical analysis

Two sample t-test was used to determine baseline differences between the normal weight and overweight children. A two-way repeated measure ANOVA (with Bonferroni post hoc test) was used to compare the effect of different types of training on heart rate, energy intake [total and normalized to body weight (energy/kg)] and the relative consumption of protein, fat, and carbohydrate in the normal weight and overweight children. Exercise type served as the within group, and weight as the between group factor. Statistical significance was taken at $p < 0.05$. Chi-square test was used to determine the differences in the number of participants at each group that increased their caloric intake per kg body weight by more than 5%. Data are presented as mean ± standard deviation (SD).

11.3 RESULTS

Anthropometric characteristics of the study participants are shown in Table 11.1. As defined, body weight, BMI and BMI percentile were significantly greater in the overweight children. There was no age, gender or pubertal status difference between the groups.

Table 11.1. Anthropometric characteristics of the study participants (*p<0.0001).

	Normal weight (n=22)	Overweight (n=22)
Age (years)	9.4±0.3	9.1±0.6
Gender (Female/male)	17/5	15/7
Height (cm)	136.1±1.3	139.4±2.5
Weight (kg)	31.7±1.1	46.9±2.2*
BMI (kg/m^2)	17.0±0.4	23.9±0.6*
BMI percentile (%)	53.2±5.0	95.2±0.8*
Pubertal stage (#)	1.3±0.1	1.3±0.1

In both groups, heart rate was significantly higher during the outdoor aerobic and swimming session compared to the resistance session and control session. In both groups heart rate during the resistance session was higher compared to the control session. There were no significant differences in mean heart rate between the normal weight and the overweight children during any of the four sessions.

In the normal weight children, total caloric intake was reduced following exercise. This difference reached statistical significance only following the resistance type exercise (19.4+1.7 versus 14.0±1.4 kcal/kg in control and resistance exercise, respectively; p<0.008). The different types of exercise were associated with increased relative consumption of carbohydrate and decreased consumption of fat. In contrast, in the overweight children, total caloric intake was increased following exercise. This increase reached statistical significance following swimming (18.5±1.5 versus 23.0±2.4 kcal/kg in control and swimming exercise, respectively; p<0.02). All types of exercise lead to a significant increase in the relative consumption of proteins in the overweight children. The total caloric intake was significantly greater in the overweight children following the swimming practice (15.9±1.6 versus 23.0±2.4 kcal/kg in normal weight and overweight, respectively; p<0.04).

11.4 DISCUSSION

We found that the immediate effect of exercise on macronutrient choices differ significantly between normal weight and overweight pre-pubertal children. As hypothesized, in the normal weight children, total energy intake was reduced following resistance-type exercise. Moreover, the different types of exercise were associated with increased relative consumption of carbohydrate and decreased consumption of fat in the normal weight children. In contrast, overweight children significantly increased their energy intake following the swimming exercise session. All types of exercise (i.e. resistance, aerobic and swimming) lead to a significant increase in the relative consumption of proteins in the overweight children (Figure 11.1). Finally, the total energy intake was significantly greater in the overweight children following the swimming practice.

Normal Weight

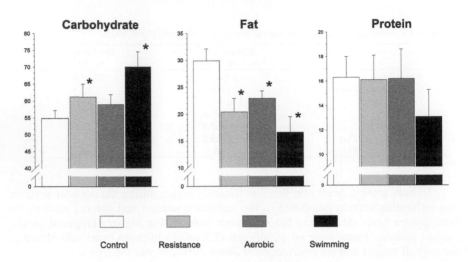

Overweight

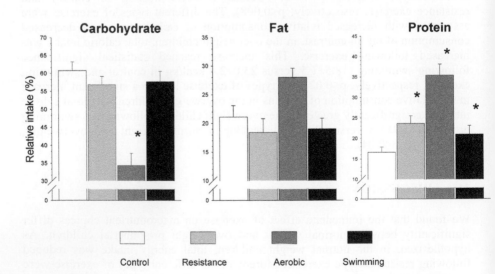

Figure 11.1. The relative consumption of carbohydrate, fat and proteins following the different types of exercise in the normal weight and overweight children. * p<0.05 compared to the no exercise session.

The increase in energy intake in the overweight children was mainly due to a significant increase in protein consumption following each of the exercise sessions. The mechanism for the differences between normal weight and overweight children and for the post-exercise increase in energy and protein intake in obese children is not known. However, we previously demonstrated that the growth hormone and catecholamine response to exercise is attenuated and the dopamine response is almost completely blunted in obese compared to normal weight children and adolescents (Eliakim *et al.*, 2006). Therefore, we can only hypothesize that the blunted growth hormone and catecholamine response and the absence of dopamine response to exercise lead to reduced carbohydrate and fat utilization during exercise, and as a result to a greater protein utilization. Increased protein utilization may explain why previous resistance training studies in children, demonstrated that elevated BMI was associated with reduced training effect on muscle mass and strength (Falk *et al.*, 2002). This may explain why in the obese children appetite was not suppressed following exercise, and protein intake was increased immediately after all types of exercise.

In summary, our data suggest that macronutrient intake and preferences in response to exercise are different in normal weight and obese children. Normal weight children decrease their total energy intake and fat consumption and increase their carbohydrate intake, while overweight children increase their total energy and protein intake, particularly following swimming. Understanding the complicated relationship between different types of exercise, appetite and food choices may help us to optimize exercise training interventions for this unique population, and to select the best exercise protocols to achieve the desired energy balance. Further studies are needed to explore the longer effect of a single exercise and the effect of exercise training interventions on appetite and food choices in children, and in particular in obese children.

11.5 REFERENCES

Dietz, W.H., 2004, Overweight in childhood and adolescence. *New England Journal of Medicine,* **350**, pp. 855–857.

Eliakim, A., Nemet, D., Zaldivar, F., McMurray, R.G., Culler, F.L., Galassetti, P. and Cooper, D.M., 2006,. Reduced exercise-associated response of the GH-IGF-I axis and catecholamines in obese children and adolescents. *Journal of Applied Physiology,* **100**, pp. 1630–1637.

Falk, B., Sadres, E., Constantini, N., Zigel, L., Lidor, R. and Eliakim, A., 2002, The association between adiposity and the response to resistance training among pre- and early- pubertal boys. *Journal of Pediatric Endocrinology and Metabolism,* **15**, pp. 597–606.

Verger, P., Lanteaume, M.T. and Louis-Sylvestre, J., 1992, Human intake and choice of foods at intervals after exercise. *Appetite,* **18**, pp. 93–99.

'Fatmax' and the Lactate Response to Exercise in Adolescents

K. Tolfrey[1], and A.M. Batterham[2]

[1]Loughborough University, UK; [2]Teesside University, UK

12.1 INTRODUCTION

Exercise intensity is the primary determinant of substrate oxidation (van Loon *et al.*, 2001) and several studies have examined this relationship in young people (Aucouturier *et al.*, 2008). The majority of studies suggest that young people tend to utilise more fat, and less carbohydrate, than adults when completing the same exercise tasks (Riddell, 2008). The exercise intensity at which maximal fat oxidation rate occurs has been dubbed the Fatmax (Jeukendrup and Achten, 2001) and there has been a resurgent interest in this parameter, particularly in obese boys (e.g., Lazzer *et al.*, 2007; Zunquin *et al.*, 2009). However, despite this interest, the control mechanisms for the rapid decline in fat oxidation at exercise intensities above Fatmax are not completely understood. As exercise intensity increases, it has been suggested that carnitine palmitoyltransferase I (CPT-I) activity, a rate-limiting enzyme in the transfer of long chain fatty acids (LCFA) into the mitochondria, is inhibited (Coyle *et al.*, 1997). Reductions in pH in *in vitro* studies with human skeletal muscle (Starritt *et al.*, 2000) and availability of free carnitine (van Loon *et al.*, 2001), the principle substrate for CPT I, are leading mechanisms thought to limit CPT I activity and fat oxidation. Subsequently, the relationship between Fatmax and the blood (plasma) lactate response to incremental exercise has been examined in adults (Achten and Jeukendrup, 2004). This study concluded that Fatmax and the intensity at which plasma [lactate] increased above baseline (LIAB) coincide at the group level, but it failed to account for between parameter variation at the individual participant level. In light of these findings, the aim of the current study was to determine whether the Fatmax and LIAB coincide in a mixed-sex group of adolescents. Other than the population, a novel feature of this study was the use of statistical procedures that account for both systematic bias and random error of the measurements.

12.2   METHODS

Complete data were available for 11 girls and 8 boys (mean (SD) age 13.9(0.3) y) at the conclusion of the study. Informed consent was provided for all participants. The LIAB and Fatmax were determined using a discontinuous, incremental cycling protocol with 8 x 3 min exercise stages following an 11 h fast. Cycling peak $\dot{V}O_2$ was determined separately after breakfast and a 45 min rest. Fat oxidation was estimated using standard stoichiometry (Frayn, 1983) from the expired air samples collected in the final minute of each 3 min exercise stage. Individual second order polynomial models of % peak $\dot{V}O_2$ against absolute fat oxidation (mg·min^{-1}) were used to identify Fatmax for each participant. Fatmax was also expressed relative to % peak heart rate (HR).

Fatmax and LIAB, expressed either as % peak $\dot{V}O_2$ or % peak HR, were compared using a nonparametric version of the limits of agreement method (Bland and Altman, 1999). Prior to data analysis, we defined the threshold for the minimum clinically important difference (MCID) between the Fatmax and LIAB parameters as ±8%. A tolerance limit of ±8% for agreement between Fatmax and LIAB is an acceptable empirical threshold for the smallest important difference in the absence of a more robust clinical or physiological anchor. We calculated the proportion of differences separately for girls and boys falling within our pre-defined MCID. Confidence intervals (90%) for this estimate were derived from a bootstrap resampling technique (Efron and Tibshirani, 1993). Systematic bias was evaluated by calculating the mean difference between parameters for boys and girls separately, then averaging to provide a point estimate of the population bias between parameters. We derived confidence intervals (90%) for this bias using the nonparametric bootstrap resampling technique described above.

12.3   RESULTS

The mean(SD) Fatmax occurred at 35(6)% peak $\dot{V}O_2$ which corresponded to 58(9)% peak HR. The LIAB of 0.98(0.21) mmol·L^{-1} occurred at 39(7)% peak $\dot{V}O_2$ which corresponded to 63(9)% peak HR. For Fatmax and LIAB as a percentage of peak $\dot{V}O_2$, the estimated population proportion with between-method agreement within ±8% was 0.76 (90% CI 0.60 to 0.91) (Figure 12.1). The group mean difference between parameters (Fatmax minus LIAB) was -3.8% peak $\dot{V}O_2$ (-5.8 to -1.8%). The probability that the true (population) difference is greater than ±8% was 0.0003 which is 'almost certainly not' clinically important. When Fatmax and LIAB were expressed as a percentage of peak HR, the estimated population proportion with between-method agreement within ±8% was also 0.76 (0.60 to 0.91). The mean difference between parameters (Fatmax minus LIAB) was -4.4% peak HR (-6.6 to -2.2%). The probability that the true (population) difference is greater than ±8% was 0.004; this is 'almost certainly not' clinically important.

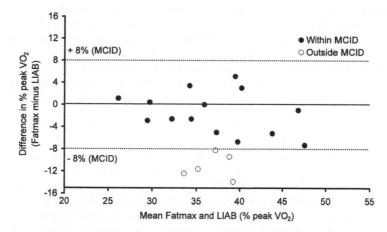

Figure 12.1. Bland-Altman plot of differences in % peak $\dot{V}O_2$ for Fatmax and LIAB against the mean of these two measurements. Closed circles (●) are the proportion of participants falling within the chosen minimum clinically important difference (MCID) of ±8% peak $\dot{V}O_2$, whereas open circles (○) are those falling outside of the MCID.

12.4 CONCLUSION

Two complementary findings emerged from this study; (i) comparison at the group level showed that Fatmax and LIAB coincide within the tolerance limit given by the MCID of ±8% peak $\dot{V}O_2$. Although the group mean differences in % peak $\dot{V}O_2$ and % peak HR would have been statistically significant when comparing Fatmax with LIAB using conventional null hypothesis testing (i.e., P≤0.05), the magnitude-based inferences indicated that the mean population differences were 'almost certainly not' clinically important. Furthermore, (ii) when considering between-parameter measurement error at the individual level, the relative exercise intensities at Fatmax and LIAB coincided in three quarters (0.76) of the adolescent girls and boys in our study. The 90% confidence intervals for this proportion showed that the agreement between the two parameters may be within the MCID in-between 6 and 9 out of 10 participants. Thus, comparisons at both the group and individual level suggest that Fatmax and the LIAB essentially coincide in adolescents. Therefore, this would appear to corroborate similar findings in adults. Further work is required where [lactate] and/or pH are manipulated in young people to examine a possible cause-effect mechanism that cannot be determined from the current study.

12.5 REFERENCES

Achten, J. and Jeukendrup, A.E., 2004, Relationship between plasma lactate concentration and fat oxidation rates over a wide range of exercise intensities. *International Journal of Sports Medicine*, **25**, pp. 32–37.

Aucouturier, J., Baker, J.S. and Duché, P., 2008, Fat and carbohydrate metabolism during submaximal exercise in children. *Sports Medicine*, **38**, pp. 213–238.

Bland, J.M. and Altman, D.G., 1999, Measuring agreement in method comparison studies. *Statistical Methods in Medical Research,* 8, pp. 135–160.

Coyle, E.F., Jeukendrup, A.E., Wagenmakers, A.J. and Saris, W.H., 1997, Fatty acid oxidation is directly regulated by carbohydrate metabolism during exercise. *American Journal of Physiology and Endocrinology and Metabolism*, **273**, pp. E268–E275.

Efron, B. and Tibshirani, R.J., 1993, *An Introduction to the Bootstrap,* (New York: Chapman & Hall), pp. 436.

Frayn, KN., 1983, Calculation of substrate oxidation rates in vivo from gaseous exchange. *Journal of Applied Physiology,* **55**, pp. 628–634.

Jeukendrup, A.E. and Achten, J., 2001, Fatmax: a new concept to optimize fat oxidation during exercise? *European Journal of Sport Science*, **1**, pp. 1–5.

Lazzer, S., Busti, C., Agosti, F., De Col, A., Pozzo, R. and Sartorio, A., 2007, Optimizing fat oxidation through exercise in severely obese Caucasian adolescents. *Clinical and Endocrinology*, **67**, pp. 582–588.

Riddell, M.C., 2008, The endocrine response and substrate utilization during exercise in children and adolescents. *Journal of Applied Physiology,* **105**, pp. 725–733.

Starritt, E.C., Howlett, R.A., Heigenhauser, G.J. and Spriet, L.L., 2000, Sensitivity of CPT I to malonyl-CoA in trained and untrained human skeletal muscle. *American Journal of Physiology and Endocrinology and Metabolism*, **278**, pp. E462–E468.

van Loon, L.J., Greenhaff, P.L., Constantin-Teodosiu, D., Saris, W.H. and Wagenmakers, A.J., 2001, The effects of increasing exercise intensity on muscle fuel utilisation in humans. *Journal of Physiology*, **536**(Pt 1), pp. 295–304.

Zunquin, G., Theunynck, D., Sesboue, B., Arhan, P., and Bougle, D., 2009, Evolution of fat oxidation during exercise in obese pubertal boys: clinical implications. *Journal of Sports Sciences*, **27**, pp. 315–318.

Influence of Pubertal Development on Ghrelin in Young Swimmers: A Longitudinal Study

T. Jürimäe[1], E. Lätt[1], K. Haljaste[1], P. Purge[1], A. Leppik[1], A. Cicchella[2], and J. Jürimäe[1]

[1]University of Tartu, Estonia; [2]University of Bologna, Italy

13.1 INTRODUCTION

Ghrelin is a peptide hormone that was discovered in 1999 as an endogenous ligand of the growth hormone (GH) – secretagogue receptor (Kojima *et al.*, 1999). Ghrelin is a regulator of a large area of endocrine and non-endocrine functions, including the influence on GH secretion, food intake and energy balance (Korbonits *et al.*, 2004). Cross-sectional studies conducted in healthy children and adolescents have found that ghrelin concentrations gradually decrease during childhood and adolescence with advancing pubertal stage (Lebenthal *et al.*, 2006).

According to our knowledge, no longitudinal studies have been performed to examine the association between ghrelin and peak oxygen consumption in young swimmers during pubertal development. Given the importance of different regulatory roles of ghrelin in energy homeostasis (Foster-Schubert *et al.*, 2004), we hypothesised that ghrelin has an independent influence on peak oxygen consumption in young male athletes.

The aim of our study was to examine the influence of regular high energy expenditure (swimming training) on ghrelin concentration in male swimmers advancing from prepubertal to pubertal maturation levels. In addition, this study examined the associations of fasting ghrelin concentration with peak oxygen consumption in young swimmers.

13.2 METHODS

13.2.1 Experimental design

The subjects of our study were 19 prepubertal male (10-12 yrs) swimmers (Tanner pubertal stage 1 on the first year). Swimmers were tested once a year during two year study period (in total three times). All testing at each time was completed during the two visits of the swimmers to the laboratory. On the first visit, a venous blood sample was taken on the morning after an overnight fast. Anthropometric parameters and peak oxygen consumption on the cycle ergometer were measured after a light breakfast. Swimmers were at the pubertal stages 2 and 3, and at the pubertal stages 3 and 4 at the second and third year measurements, respectively. Subjects' swimming training history were 2.6 ± 0.8 yrs and have been training for 7.6 ± 1.5 hrs per week for at least the last two years. All procedures were approved by the Medical Ethics Committee of the University of Tartu, Estonia and explained to the children and their parents who signed a consent form. Body height was measured with Martin metal anthropometer and body mass with a medical balance scale (A&D Instruments, UK). Body mass index (BMI) was calculated as body mass (kg) divided by body height (m^2).

13.2.2 Blood samples

A venous blood sample was taken in the morning after an overnight fast for ghrelin measurement (RIA, Linco Research, USA). The sensitivity was 93 pg/ml, the intra-assay and inter-assay CVs were < 10 and 14.7%, respectively.

13.2.3 Peak oxygen consumption

Peak oxygen consumption (l/min) was measured on an electronically braked cycle ergometer (Tunturi T8, Finland). Participants performed an initial work rate at 80 W with increments of 20 W every 2 min. At the end of the last work rate, participants were required to sprint as fast as possible for 1 min. Swimmers pedalled at a cadence of 70 ± 5 rpm, and they were actively encouraged to continue until volitional exhaustion. Gas exchange variables were measured throughout the test in breath-by-breath mode and data were stored in 10 s intervals for the measurement of oxygen consumption using portable open circuit system (MedGraphics VO200, St. Paul, USA).

13.2.4 Statistical analysis

Statistical analysis was performed using SPSS 13.0. Standard statistical methods were used to calculate mean (X) and ±SD. The differences between measurement times were tested with Friedman analysis of Variance by ranks and Wilcoxon matched-pairs signed rank test was used where post hoc analysis was relevant. Pearson correlation coefficients were used to determine the relationships between independent variables. Significance was set at p<0.05.

13.3 RESULTS

Mean anthropometrical parameters, ghrelin concentration and peak oxygen consumption of the subjects are presented in Table 13.1.

Table 13.1. Mean (±SD) physical characteristics, ghrelin concentration and peak oxygen consumption in young male swimmers (n=19).

	Year 1	Year 2	Year 3
Age (yrs)	11.4 ± 0.8	12.4 ± 0.8*	13.4 ± 0.8*#
Body height (cm)	155.0 ± 8.9	162.6 ± 9.2*	167.6 ± 8.9*#
Body weight (kg)	42.8 ± 9.2	49.3 ± 10.3*	54.9 ± 10.4*#
BMI (kg/m^2)	17.6 ± 2.3	18.6 ± 2.4*	19.4 ± 2.5*#
Ghrelin (pg/ml)	1321.8 ± 446.4	910.0 ± 343.6*	900.6 ± 339.6*
$\dot{V}O_{2peak}$ (l/min)	2.54 ± 0.45	3.07 ± 0.52*	3.14 ± 0.50*

*Significantly different from the first measurement (p<0.05)

#Significantly different from the second measurement (p<0.05)

Height, body mass and BMI increased accordingly to the pubertal development in all boys at each measurement point. Peak oxygen uptake was increased and ghrelin concentration was decreased only after the first year of measurement. Ghrelin concentration was significantly related to BMI at all three measurement times (r=-0.551 to -0.661) and $\dot{V}O_2$ peak (r=-0.482 to -0.503).

13.4 CONCLUSIONS

Circulating ghrelin levels remained relatively high also during puberty in our young swimmers compared to other studies with untrained boys (Whatmore *et al.*, 2003). In our previous study physically active girls (swimmers) had significantly higher mean plasma ghrelin levels than physically inactive girls (Jürimäe *et al.*, 2007). In our study fasting ghrelin was not correlated significantly with Tanner stages. Bellone *et al.* (2002) concluded that ghrelin was independent of pubertal status in lean children. This means that our results support the possibility that ghrelin may act independently during different stages of maturation in the presence of regular high energy expenditure in swimmers.

In conclusion, the ghrelin concentration was decreased and peak oxygen consumption increased at onset of puberty, while no further changes were seen with advancing age and pubertal stage in young male swimmers. Finally, ghrelin concentration in blood correlated negatively with peak oxygen consumption.

13.5 REFERENCES

Bellone, S., Rapa, A., Vivenza, D., Castellino, N., Petri, A., Bellone, J., Me, E., Broglio, F., Prodam, F., Ghigo, E. and Bona, G., 2002, Circulating ghrelin levels as function of gender, pubertal status and adiposity in childhood. *Journal of Endocrinological Investigation*, **25**, pp. RC13–RC15.

Foster-Schubert, K.E., Tiernan, A., Frayo, R.S., Schwartz, R.S., Rajan, K.B., Yasui, Y., Tworoger, S.S. and Cummings, D.E., 2004, Human plasma ghrelin levels increase during one-year exercise program. *Journal of Clinical Endocrinology and Metabolism*, **90**, pp. 820–825.

Jürimäe, J., Cicchella, A., Jürimäe, T., Lätt, E., Haljaste, K., Purge, P., Hamra, J. and von Duvillard, S.P., 2007, Regular physical activity influences plasma ghrelin concentration in adolescent girls. *Medicine and Science in Sports and Exercise*, **39**, pp. 1736–1741.

Kojima, M., Hosoda, H., Date, F., Nakazato, M., Matsuo, H. and Kangawa, K., 1999, Ghrelin as a growth-hormone-releasing acylated peptide from stomach. *Nature*, **402**, pp. 656–660.

Korbonits, M., Goldstone, A.P., Gueorguiev, M. and Grossman, A.B., 2004, Ghrelin- a hormone with multiple functions. *Frontiers in Neuroendocrinology*, **25**, pp. 27–68.

Lebenthal, Y., Gat-Yablonski, G., Shtaif, B., Padoa, A., Phillip, M. and Lazar, L., 2006, Effect of sex hormone administration on circulating ghrelin levels in prepubertal children. *Journal of Clinical Endocrinology and Metabolism*, **91**, pp. 328–331.

Whatmore, A.J., Hall, C.M., Jones, J., Westwood, M. and Clayton, P.E., 2003, Ghrelin concentration in healthy children and adolescents. *Clinical Endocrinology*, **59**, pp. 649–654.

Part III

Hormonal and Inflammatory Regulations

CHAPTER NUMBER 14

Anabolic Hormones and Inflammatory Markers in Elite Male and Female Adolescent Players Following Volleyball Practice

A. Eliakim[1], S. Portal[1], Z. Zadik[2], J. Rabinowitz[3], D. Adler-Portal[1], D.M. Cooper[4], F. Zaldivar[4], and D. Nemet[1]

[1]Child Health & Sport Center, Pediatric Department, Meir Medical Center, Sackler School of Medicine, Tel-Aviv University, Israel; [2]Pediatric Endocrine Unit, Kaplan Medical Center, Rehovot, Israel; [3]Bar-Ilan University, Ramat Gan, Israel; [4]Pediatric Exercise Research Center, Department of Pediatrics, University Children's Hospital, University California, Irvine, California, USA

14.1   INTRODUCTION

Extensive efforts are made in competitive sports to quantify objectively the fine balance between training intensity and athlete's tolerance. Recent reports suggest that exercise leads to a simultaneous increase of antagonistic mediators. Exercise stimulates anabolic components of the growth hormone (GH) → IGF-I (insulin-like growth factor-I) axis (Eliakim et al., 2005), and elevates catabolic pro-inflammatory cytokines such as Interlukin-6 (IL-6), IL-1 and tumor necrosis factor-α (TNF- α) as well (Nemet et al., 2002). It was suggested that evaluation of the exercise-induced changes in these circulating mediators can provide a new insight into quantification of training loads. The effect of a single exercise and/or exercise training on the GH-IGF-I axis and inflammatory cytokines was studied mainly in adults participating in individualized endurance-type sports. Only recently several studies examined the effect of supra-maximal anaerobic bout (Wingate anaerobic test) and sprint interval training on these mediators (Meckel et al., 2009, Stokes et al., 2005). Very few studies have examined the effect of training on the GH-IGF-I axis and inflammatory markers in children and adolescent elite athletes, and in team sports which are very popular in these age groups (Nemet et al., 2003). Moreover, gender-associated differences in the response of these circulating mediators to exercise training in elite athletes have not been studied thoroughly. Therefore, the purpose of this study was to evaluate the effect of a typical volleyball practice on anabolic (GH, IGF-I and testosterone) and catabolic hormones (cortisol), and inflammatory mediators (IL-6) in elite, national team level, male and female adolescent volleyball players. Volleyball use was chosen because it is a very popular team sport for both genders, and involves both aerobic and anaerobic properties.

14.2   METHODS

Twenty seven (14 males, 13 females) healthy elite, national team level Israeli junior volleyball players (age range 13.5 - 18 years, Tanner stage for pubic hair 4-5) participated in the study. All participants played in the Israeli premier junior volleyball league, belonged to the Israeli national junior volleyball team and were members of the Israeli National Academy for Gifted Athletes. The study was performed during the very early phase of the volleyball season.

14.2.1 Exercise protocol

Exercise consisted of a typical one hour volleyball practice including 20 minutes dynamic warm-up which included jogging, stretching and running drills at sub-maximal speed (up to 80% of maximal speed), and additional 20 minutes of volleyball drills. The main part of the practice included seven repetitions of seven consecutive sprints from the back of the volleyball court to the net, maximal jump and a hit of the volleyball over the net in the end of each sprint. Each repetition lasted about 1.5 minutes with one minute rest to collect the balls between repetitions.

14.2.2 Blood sampling

Hormonal measurements included circulating levels of the anabolic hormones GH, IGF-I, IGF binding protein-3 (IGFBP-3) and testosterone and the catabolic hormone cortisol. Measurements of inflammatory mediators included the pro-inflammatory markers IL-6, and the anti-inflammatory marker IL-1 receptor antagonist (IL-1ra). Blood samples were collected before and immediately after the practice. All female participants had regular menses, and blood samples were collected during the early follicular phase of their menstrual cycle (first five days of the cycle).

14.2.3 Statistical analysis

Two sample t-test was used to compare baseline and post exercise anthropometric, fitness and hormonal levels between male and female players. Repeated measures ANOVA was used to assess the effect of exercise on circulating components of the GH-IGF-I axis and inflammatory mediators with time serving as the within group factor and gender as the between group factor. Data are presented as mean ± SEM. Significance was set at an alpha level of $p \leq 0.05$.

14.3 RESULTS

Exercise led to significant increases in GH (0.2 ± 0.1 to 2.7 ± 0.7 and 1.7 ± 0.5 to 6.4 ± 1.4 ng/ml, in males and females respectively, $p<0.05$ for both), testosterone (6.1 ± 0.9 to 7.3 ± 1.0 and 2.4 ± 0.6 to 3.3 ± 0.7 ng/ml, in males and females respectively, $p<0.05$ for both), and IL-6 (1.1 ± 0.6 to 3.1 ± 1.5 and 1.2 ± 0.5 to 2.5 ± 1.1 pg/ml, in males and females respectively, $p<0.002$ for both). Exercise had no significant effect on IGF-I, IGFBP-3, cortisol and IL1ra levels.

In the female players baseline levels of GH and cortisol were significantly higher and testosterone levels significantly lower compared to male players. Levels of testosterone were significantly lower in the female players at the end of exercise as well. There was no significant difference in the volleyball practice-induced changes in GH, testosterone and IL-6 levels between genders.

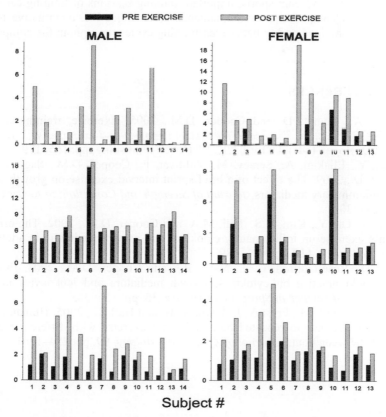

Figure 14.1. The effects of single volleyball training on GH, testosterone and IL-6 in elite adolescent male and female players.

* Significant difference between males and females; # Significant difference from baseline levels for both genders.

14.4   CONCLUSION

Changes in GH and testosterone following the volleyball practice suggest exercise-related anabolic adaptations. The increase in IL-6 may indicate its important role in muscle tissue repair. Despite significantly higher GH levels in the females, and higher testosterone levels in the males, there were no significant gender-related differences in the hormonal and inflammatory response to the volleyball practice. This suggests that testosterone, despite its very low levels, can be used as an exercise-associated anabolic marker even in female athletes.

The results indicate that changes in the anabolic-catabolic hormonal balance and in circulating inflammatory cytokines can be used by the athlete and/or his coach to gauge the training intensity also in team sports such as volleyball. It is clear that these responses can not be used as a marker for every practice, unless future techniques will provide immediate results (like the current ability to assess lactate levels). However, the response of these hormones can be used occasionally in different types of team sports, important training sessions or training camps, or prior to main competitions or tournaments, as an objective, quantitative tool to monitor training load and to better plan training cycles throughout the competitive season.

14.5   REFERENCES

Eliakim, A., Nemet, D. and Cooper, D.M., 2005, Exercise, training and the GH→IGF-I axis. In: *The endocrine system in sports and exercise.* W.J. Kraemer and A.D. Rogol, (eds), Oxford, UK, Blackwell Publishing, pp. 165–179.

Meckel, Y., Eliakim, A., Seraev, M., Zaldivar, F., Cooper, D.M., Sagiv M. and Nemet, D., 2009, The effect of a brief sprint interval exercise on growth factors and inflammatory mediators. *Journal of Strength and Conditioning Research, 23*, pp. 225–230.

Nemet, D., Oh, Y., Kim, H.S., Hill, M.A. and Cooper, D.M., 2002, The effect of intense exercise on inflammatory cytokines and growth mediators in adolescent boys. *Pediatrics, 110*, pp. 681–689.

Nemet, D., Rose-Gottron, C.M., Mills, P.J. and Cooper, D.M., 2003, Effect of water polo practice on cytokines, growth mediators and leukocytes in girls. *Medicine and Science in Sports and Exercise, 35*, pp. 356–363.

Stokes, K., Nevill, M., Frystyk, J., Lakomy, H. and Hall, G., 2005, Human growth hormone response to repeated bouts of sprint exercise with different recovery periods between bouts. *Journal of Applied Physiology, 99*, pp. 254–1261.

Effect of Continuous and Intermittent Exercise on Immune Cell Responses in Children with and without a Chronic Inflammatory Disease

J. Obeid[1], H.E. Ploeger[1], T. Nguyen[1], T. Takken[1,2], and
B.W. Timmons[1]

[1]Children's Exercise and Nutrition Centre, McMaster University, Hamilton, ON,
Canada; [2]Wilhelmina Children's Hospital, University Medical Center Utrecht, the
Netherlands

15.1 INTRODUCTION

Chronic inflammatory diseases are characterized by persistent local and systemic inflammation as seen in Crohn's disease (CD), cystic fibrosis (CF) and juvenile idiopathic arthritis (JIA). Historically, physical inactivity was prescribed as an essential component of therapy for children with chronic inflammatory disease – the rationale for which was that inflammatory conditions are best treated by rest (Bar-Or and Rowland, 2004; Eising and Soules, 1964). The evidence now demonstrates that exercise tolerance can be associated with the general health of these patients (Nixon *et al.*, 1992; Takken *et al.*, 2008). In fact, children with a chronic inflammatory disease are often encouraged by their physicians and physiotherapists to maintain and/or increase levels of physical activity; however, very little advice is given as to what the type, duration, or intensity of this exercise should be (The Arthritis Society of Canada, 2009). This may be attributable to the fact that to date, very few studies have examined the effect of acute exercise on inflammation in chronic inflammatory disease (Ploeger *et al.*, 2009).

In healthy children, a single bout of exercise is known to induce transient increases in the very same inflammatory markers that are pathological in chronic inflammatory disease (Timmons, 2005; Timmons *et al.*, 2006). Much less is known about this issue in children with a chronic inflammatory disease, but a clearer understanding of exercise and inflammation in this population would help inform evidence-based exercise prescription. As such, the aim of this study was to examine the effect of two distinct, yet clinically relevant forms of acute exercise on immune cells, and to compare these responses in children with and without chronic inflammatory diseases.

15.2   METHODS

Sixteen children (mean (SD), age: 13.8 (2.3) years) participated in this study, among these were 10 children diagnosed with CD, 5 with CF and 1 with JIA who composed the patient group. Sixteen children without a disease (age: 13.3 (2.4) years) were also tested and matched with the patients by biological age (years from peak height velocity) (Mirwald *et al.*, 2002); these children composed the control group.

Peak aerobic mechanical power (PP) was determined in session 1 using the McMaster Progressive All-Out Continuous Protocol. In sessions 2 and 3, children performed either: a) moderate intensity, continuous exercise (MICE) consisting of 2x30-min bouts of cycling at 50%PP, or b) high intensity, intermittent exercise (HIIE) consisting of 6 sets of 4x15-sec bouts of cycling at 100%PP. These sessions were performed in a counterbalanced fashion. Blood was drawn at rest, at the mid-point (EX-MID) and end of exercise (EX-END), and after 30 (REC-30) and 60 min (REC-60) of recovery to determine changes in neutrophil, lymphocyte and monocyte counts.

Two-way ANOVAs were performed to compare the response to exercise between the controls and patients. Statistical significance was set at $p \leq 0.05$. Tukey's Honestly Significant Differences test was used to further examine significant differences.

15.3   RESULTS

15.3.1 Neutrophils

Absolute neutrophil counts in patients were significantly higher at each sampling time point when compared with controls in both MICE and HIIE ($p < 0.05$). When looking at changes from rest, MICE resulted in significant increases in neutrophil counts at EX-END, REC-30 and REC-60 in both patients and controls, with no significant differences between the groups ($p > 0.05$). Similarly, no differences were seen between patients and controls for HIIE where neutrophil counts were significantly increased at EX-MID and EX-END but returned to baseline levels by REC-30 (Figure 15.1).

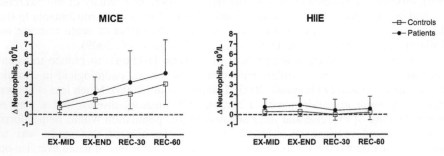

Figure 15.1. Changes from rest in neutrophils during and following MICE and HIIE.

15.3.2 Lymphocytes

Absolute lymphocyte counts tended to be lower in patients compared with controls at all time points in MICE and HIIE. Both MICE and HIIE induced significant increases in lymphocyte counts at EX-MID and EX-END in patients and controls, returning to resting levels by REC-30 (Figure 15.2). The only difference between groups occurred at EX-END in the MICE protocol where patients demonstrated a significantly lower change from rest compared with controls (mean (SD), 0.55 (0.44) vs. 0.96 (0.94) x 10^9/L, p <0.005).

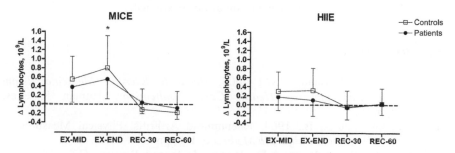

Figure 15.2. Changes from rest in lymphocytes during and following MICE and HIIE.

15.3.3 Monocytes

Absolute monocyte counts were significantly greater in patients compared with controls at REC-30 and REC-60 for MICE, while patients and controls were similar for HIIE. Changes in monocyte counts from rest were not significantly different between groups in MICE and HIIE (Figure 15.3). Exercise induced a significant increase in monocyte counts in MICE, which remained significantly elevated into REC-60, while HIIE resulted in increased monocytes counts at EX-MID and EX-END, returning to baseline by REC-30.

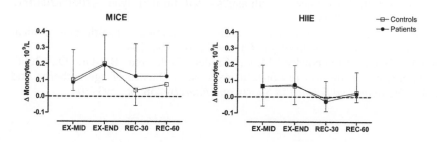

Figure 15.3. Changes from rest in monocytes during and following MICE and HIIE.

15.4   CONCLUSION

These preliminary data suggest that while the absolute neutrophil and monocyte counts tended to be elevated in patients, the response to exercise (i.e., change from rest) was similar between groups. Moreover, MICE appeared to induce a greater change in immune cell counts compared with HIIE.

Future work needs to assess whether differences exist in the immune cell responses to exercise in the individual conditions of CD, CF and JIA. Furthermore, the effect of MICE and HIIE on inflammatory markers related to disease pathology (i.e., interleukin-6, tumour necrosis factor alpha) and growth factors (i.e., growth hormone, insulin-like growth factor 1) should be examined.

15.5   REFERENCES

Bar-Or, O. and Rowland, T.W., 2004, *Pediatric Exercise Medicine: From Physiologic Principles to Health Care Applications*, Human Kinetics, Champaign, IL.

Eising, L. and Soules, B., 1964, Rheumatoid Arthritis: Physical Measures in Treatment of Children. *California Medicine,* **100**, pp. 340–342.

Mirwald, R.L., Baxter-Jones, A.D., Bailey, D.A. and Beunen, G.P., 2002, An assessment of maturity from anthropometric measurements. *Medicine and Science in Sport and Exercise*, **34**, pp. 689–694.

Nixon, P.A., Orenstein, D.M., Kelsey, S.F. and Doershuk, C.F., 1992, The prognostic value of exercise testing in patients with cystic fibrosis. *New England Journal of Medicine*, **327**, pp. 1785–1788.

Ploeger, H.E., Takken, T., de Greef, M.H. G. and Timmons, B.W., 2009, The effects of acute and chronic exercise on inflammatory markers in children and adults with a chronic inflammatory disease: a systematic review. *Exercise Immunology Review*, **15**, pp. 6–41.

Takken, T., van Brussel, M., Engelbert, R.H., Van Der, N.J., Kuis, W. and Helders, P.J., 2008, Exercise therapy in juvenile idiopathic arthritis. *Cochrane Database Systematic Review*, CD005954.

The Arthritis Society of Canada, 2009 Juvenile Arthritis. http://www.arthritis.ca/splash/default.asp?s=1&ReturnUrl=types%20of%20arthritis:childhood, 4-28-2008.

Timmons, B.W., 2005, Paediatric exercise immunology: health and clinical applications. *Exercise Immunology Review*, **11**, pp. 108–144.

Timmons, B.W., Tarnopolsky, M.A., Snider, D.P. and Bar-Or, O., 2006, Immunological changes in response to exercise: influence of age, puberty, and gender. *Medicine and Science in Sports and Exercise*, **38**, pp. 293–304.

Taekwondo Fighting Simulation and Hormonal Response in Elite Adolescent Fighters

R. Pilz-Burstein[1], Y. Ashkenazi[2], Y. Yaakobovitz[2], Y. Cohen[2], L. Zigel[1], D. Nemet[3], N. Shamash[2], and A. Eliakim[3]

[1]The Ribstein Center for Research and Sports Medicine Sciences, Wingate Institute, Netanya, Israel; [2]Israel School Sports Association; [3]Child Health & Sports Center, Pediatric Department, Meir Medical Center, Sackler School of Medicine, Tel-Aviv University, Israel

16.1   INTRODUCTION

Taekwondo was recognized as an Olympic sport in the 2000 Sidney Olympic games. Taekwondo requires both anaerobic and aerobic capabilities and fights are characterized by discontinious, explosive, rapid movements performed mainly by the lower part of the athlete's body.

Very little is known about the involvement of adolescent male and female athletes in Taekwondo, and about their energy demands and endocrine responses during training and competition. Understanding of the physiological demands and hormonal responses of athletes to a single exercise, during longer training periods and during competition plays a key role in the development of a sport-specific conditioning program. Recent reports suggest that exercise may lead to a simultaneous increase of both anabolic and catabolic mediators (Eliakim et al., 2005, Nemet et al., 2002).

Therefore, the aim of the present study was to assess the hormonal responses during a fighting simulation day in elite, national team level, adolescent, male and female, taekwondo athletes. We hypothesized that the fighting simulation day will be associated with increases in the anabolic hormones IGF-I and testosterone levels, and the catabolic hormone cortisol.

16.2   METHODS

Twenty athletes (10 boys, 10 girls; mean age: 14.4 ± 1.0 y.o.) who belong to the "Golden Hope" Israeli taekwondo project participated in the study. Participants train 1.5 hours per day, 5 days a week, and had a training experience of $4 - 7$ years. The study was performed prior to the competition season, at peak training level.

16.2.1 Fighting simulation day

The fighting simulation day included three fights for each participant. The length of each fight was eight minutes (3 rounds, 2 minutes each, separated by one minute of rest). The rest between fights was 30 minutes. During these 30 minutes, athletes were passive for 25 minutes and then performed light warmup (mainly taekwondo drills) during the five minutes prior to the following fight. This resting protocol is used regularly by the taekwondo fighters during competition.

16.2.2 Blood sampling

Blood samples for anabolic (IGF-I, LH, FSH, estradiol and testosterone) and catabolic hormones (cortisol) were collected before the first and immediately after the third fight.

16.2.3 Statistical analysis

Unpaired t-test was used to compare baseline anthropometric and hormonal differences between male and female taekwondo fighters. Repeated measures ANOVA was used to assess the effect of exercise on lactate, IGF-I, LH, FSH, testosterone, estradiol and cortisol with time serving as the within group factor and gender as the between group factor. Data are presented as mean ± SD. Significance was taken at $p \leq 0.05$.

16.3   RESULTS

The fighting simulation practice led to significant ($p < 0.05$) decreases in IGF-I (males: -27.1±25.6, females: -22.4±36.3 ng/ml), LH (males: -0.7±1.2, females: -2.3±3.3 mU/L) and FSH (males: -0.9±0.5, females: -1.5±1.1 mU/L), and to a significant increase ($p < 0.05$) in cortisol (males: 3.4±7.3, females: 1.1±5.7 mcg/dL) in both genders. Fighting simulation decreases in testosterone (males: -1.9±1.6, females: -0.02±0.06 ng/ml), and free androgen index (males: -20.1±21.5, females: -0.3±0.5) were significant ($p < 0.05$) only in male fighters (Figure 16.1).

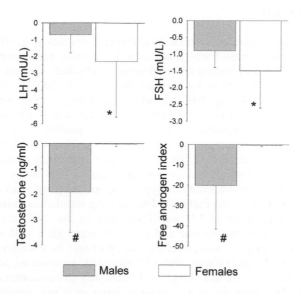

Figure 16.1. Gender-related changes in LH, FSH, testosterone and free androgen index (FAI) following the fighting simulation day. Decreases in LH and FSH were significant in both genders. Decreases of testosterone and FAI were significant only in the male taekwondo fighters (# $p<0.01$).

There was a significant increase in the cortisol/testosterone ration in both genders. This increase was significantly greater among male fighters (Figure 16.2). Exercise had no significant effect on estradiol and sex-hormone binding globulins.

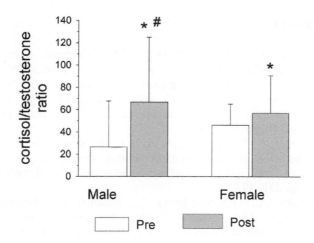

Figure 16.2. Changes in the cortisol/testosterone ratio in male and female taekwondo fighters. (*$p<0.01$ for within group, #$p<0.05$ for male versus female difference).

16.4　CONCLUSION

Previous studies demonstrated increase in anabolic hormones (e.g. GH and IGF-I) in response to short exercise training sessions. In contrast, prolonged and intense exercise sessions [1.5 h of intense soccer practice in children (Scheett *et al.*, 2002), or 1.5 h of wrestling practice in adolescents (Nemet *et al.*, 2002)] were associated with decreases in circulating IGF-I levels. Interestingly, these sessions were associated with increases in proinflammatory cytokines, and it was suggested that the increase in these proinflammatory cytokines mediated the decrease in circulating IGF-I. In the present study, the length of exercise was relatively short (3 fights, 6 min each, separated by 30 min of rest). Yet, it is possible that the combination of physiological and emotional stress of the taekwondo fighting simulation training led to the catabolic-type hormonal response (decreased IGF-I and testosterone and increased cortisol). The fighting simulation training was also associated with a decrease in LH and FSH, and in the male athletes with a concomitant decrease in testosterone and free androgen index, with no change in SHBG. The results suggest, therefore, that the decrease in testosterone and free androgen index in the males was centrally mediated. In contrast, in the female athletes, despite the decrease in LH and FSH, there was no concomitant decrease in estradiol levels. The cause for these gender differences is not clearly understood. Overall, these results are consistent with previous reports (Suay *et al.*, 1999) suggesting that while testosterone usually increases following a single exercise, the combination of physiological and psychological strain in a competition, and as shown in the present study, also in competition simulation, may lead to central suppression of testosterone level. Finally, the results suggest that changes in the anabolic-catabolic hormonal balance can be used occasionally in different types of individual fighting sports, during important training sessions and training camps, or prior to main competitions or tournaments, as an objective tool to monitor the training load and to better plan training cycles throughout the competitive season.

16.5　REFERENCES

Eliakim, A., Nemet, D. and Cooper, D.M., 2005, Exercise, training and the GH→IGF-I axis. In: *The endocrine system in sports and exercise.* W.J. Kraemer and A.D. Rogol, eds. Oxford, UK, Blackwell Publishing, pp. 165–179.

Nemet, D., Oh, Y., Kim, H.S., Hill, M.A. and Cooper, D.M., 2002, The effect of intense exercise on inflammatory cytokines and growth mediators in adolescent boys. *Pediatrics*, **110**, pp. 681–689.

Scheett, T.P., Nemet, D., Stoppani, J., Maresh, C.M., Newcomb, R. and Cooper, D.M., 2002, The effect of endurance-type exercise training on growth mediators and inflammatory cytokines in pre-pubertal and early pubertal males. *Pediatric Research*, **52**, pp. 491–497.

Suay, F., Salvador, A., Gonzalez-Bono, E., Sanchis, C., Martinez, M. and Martinez-Sanchis, S., 1999, Effects of competition and its outcome on serum testosterone, cortisol and prolactin. *Psychoneuroendocrinology*, **24**, pp. 551–566.

Bone Mineral Values, Insulin-Like Growth Factor-1, and Sex Hormones in Adolescent Female Athletes

R. Gruodyte[1,2], J. Jürimäe[1], M. Saar[1], and T. Jürimäe[1]

[1]University of Tartu, Estonia; [2]Lithuanian Academy of Physical Education, Kaunas, Lithuania

17.1 INTRODUCTION

The pubertal growth spurt accounts for about 20% of final adult height and 50% of adult peak bone mass (Wei and Gregory, 2009). Bone mass accrual during puberty is more dependable on sexual maturation than chronological age, and effects of sex hormones on the growing skeleton are associated with the osteoporosis later in life (Manolagas et al., 2002). One of the most effective osteoporosis prevention strategies may be maximising bone mineral content (BMC) during growing years by adopting weight-bearing physical activity in childhood and adolescence (French et al., 2000). High impact activities such as gymnastics, promote bone mineral accrual to a greater extent than low-impact activities such as swimming (Duncan et al., 2002). Bone mineral development in girls may be especially promoted by the increase of estrogen and insulin-like growth factor I (IGF-1) levels (MacKelvie et al., 2002). Several studies have investigated IGF-axis and sex hormone levels in relation with pubertal development and physical activity (van Coeverden et al., 2002). The positive association that exists between estradiol and bone turnover markers in early puberty disappears in late puberty and is also observed for IGF-1 (van Coeverden et al., 2002). Increasing sex hormones also increase IGF-1 levels that affect bone growth (Kanbur-Öksüz et al., 2004).

The aim of this study was to determine the relationships of bone mineral density (BMD) and BMC at femoral neck and lumbar spine with IGF-1, IGF binding protein-3 (IGFBP-3) and sex hormones in pubertal female athletes.

17.2 METHODS

The participants were 80 healthy adolescent girls aged 13-15 years. Athletic girls were rhythmic gymnasts (n = 23) and swimmers (n = 24) who have participated in their selected sports at least for the last two years. Control group (n = 33) consisted of the girls who took part only in compulsory physical education classes at school.

This study was approved by the Medical Ethics Committee of the University of Tartu (Estonia).

BMD and BMC at femoral neck and lumbar spine were measured using DXA. Venous blood samples to determine the concentration of IGF-1, IGFBP-3 and estradiol were drawn after an overnight fasting at early follicular phase and analysed in duplicate on Immulite 2000 (DPC, Los Angeles, CA, USA).

Statistical analysis was performed with SPSS 15.0 for Windows (USA). Means and standard deviations (±SD) were determined. A one-way analysis of variance (ANOVA) and Tukey *post hoc* test were used to establish the differences between the groups. Pearson's product moment correlation was used to examine relationships between parameters. Partial correlation analysis was used to examine these relationships after controlling for age, body height, and body mass (Wang *et al.*, 2004). The effect of IGF-1, IGFBP-3 and estradiol to the BMD and BMC was analysed by stepwise multiple regression analysis. The level of significance was conducted at p<0.05.

17.3   RESULTS

Mean anthropometrical and bone parameters and blood concentrations of IGF-1, IGFBP-3 and estradiol are presented on Table 17.1.

BMD values in femoral neck in rhythmic gymnasts group were higher compared with swimmers and controls. There were no significant differences between groups in measured hormones (see Table 17.1).

After adjusting for age, body height, and body mass, the relationships between BMD variables, IGF-1, and IGF-1/IGFBP-3 remained significant (r=0.46–0.60; p<0.05) in rhythmic gymnasts group but not in swimmers or controls. BMD at femoral neck and lumbar spine were also related to estradiol levels (r=0.45–0.60; p<0.05) only in rhythmic gymnast group. Only BMC at femoral neck remained associated with IGF-1/IGFBP-3 molar ratio in rhythmic gymnasts group after adjusting for age, body height, and body mass.

Table 17.1. Mean (±SD) anthropometrical parameters, bone mineral density (BMD), bone mineral content (BMC) and blood hormones in rhythmic gymnasts, swimmers and control group.

	Rhythmic gymnasts (n=23)	Swimmers (n=24)	Controls (n=33)
Age (yrs)	14.3 ± 1.0	13.7 ± 1.2[a]	14.2 ± 1.1
Body height (cm)	163.8 ± 6.7	164.2 ± 6.8	163.3 ± 6.5
Body mass (kg)	52.4 ± 8.9	55.4 ± 9.2	55.2 ± 8.1
BMI (kg/m^2)	19.4 ± 2.4	20.5 ± 2.9	20.6 ± 2.4
BMD, femoral neck (g/cm^2)	1.13 ± 0.15	1.01 ± 0.11[b]	1.01 ± 0.11[b]
BMD, lumbar spine (g/cm^2)	1.12 ± 0.11	1.08 ± 0.13	1.08 ± 0.13
BMC, femoral neck (g)	4.9 ± 0.7	4.6 ± 9.9	4.7 ± 0.7
BMC, lumbar spine (g)	44.5 ± 8.2	41.6 ± 9.9	41.4 ± 7.9
IGF-1(µg/l)	443.2 ± 104.9	463.7 ± 138.6	419.2 ± 144.9
IGFBP-3 (mg/l)	6.0 ± 0.7	5.9 ± 0.7	5.8 ± 0.9
IGF-1/IGFBP-3 molar ratio	0.27 ± 0.06	0.28 ± 0.07	0.26 ± 0.07
Estradiol (pmol/l)	67.7 ± 35.2	108.0 ± 91.4	103.1 ± 134.5

a – statistically different from rhythmic gymnasts and controls (p<0.05)
b – statistically different from rhythmic gymnasts (p<0.05)

17.4 CONCLUSIONS

The results of this study indicate the specificity of the rhythmic gymnasts (very high impact sport event) compared with swimmers (very low impact sport event) and controls. In rhythmic gymnasts, the relationship of femoral neck and lumbar spine BMD with IGF-1 and estradiol remained significant even after adjusting for age, body height, and body mass. In our study, estradiol levels had a significant relationship with femoral neck (r=0.60) and lumbar spine (r=0.45) BMD in rhythmic gymnast group only. The same associations were revealed after adjusting for the age, body height, and body mass. Estradiol is positively associated with the total volumetric BMD in pubertal girls, it was found to account for only 5.2% of the variance in total volumetric BMD (Wang *et al.*, 2004). However, rhythmic gymnasts, who had the highest femoral neck BMD had the lowest estradiol levels (see Table 17.1). Probably their hypoestragonism was partly compensated by engaging in frequent high impact loading.

We conclude that BMD correlated with IGF-1 and estradiol in pubertal rhythmic gymnasts, compared with swimmers and controls.

17.5 REFERENCES

Duncan, C.S., Blimkie, C.J.R., Cowell, C.T., Burke, S.T., Briody, J.N. and Howman-Giles, R., 2002, Bone mineral density in adolescent female athletes: relationship to exercise type and muscle strength. *Medicine and Science in Sports and Exercise*, **34**, pp. 286–294.

French, S.A., Fulkerson, J.A. and Story, M., 2000, Increasing weight-bearing physical activity and calcium intake for bone mass growth in children and adolescents: a review of intervention trials. *Preventive Medicine*, **31**, pp. 722–731.

Kanbur-Öksüz, N., Derman, O. and Kinik, E., 2004, Correlation of sex steroids with IGF-1 and IGFBP-3 during different pubertal stages. *Turkish Journal of Pediatry*, **46**, pp. 315–321.

MacKelvie, K.J., Khan, K.M. and McKay, H.A., 2002, Is there a critical period for bone response to weight-bearing exercise in children and adolescence? A systematic review. *British Journal of Sports Medicine*, **36**, pp. 250–257.

Manolagas, S.C., Kousteni, S. and Jilka, R.L., 2002, Sex steroids and bone. *Recent Progress in Hormone Research*, **57**, pp. 385–409.

van Coeverden, S.C.C.M., Netelenbos, J.C., Ridder, C.M., Roos, J.C., Popp-Snijders, C. and Delemarre-van de Waal, H.A., 2002, Bone metabolism markers and bone mass in healthy pubertal boys and girls. *Clinical Endocrinology*, **57**, pp. 107–116.

Wang, Q., Nicholson, P.H.F., Suuriniemi, M., Lyytikäinen, A., Helkala, E., Alen, M., Suominen, H. and Cheng, S., 2004, Relationships of sex hormone to bone geometric properties and mineral density in early pubertal girls. *Journal of Clinical Endocrinology and Metabolism*, **89**, 1, pp. 698–1703.

Wei, C. and Gregory, J.W., 2009, Physiology of normal growth. *Paediatric Child Health*, **19**, pp. 236–240.

Anaerobic Exercise and Salivary Cortisol, Testosterone and Immunoglobulin (a) in 15-16 Year Old Boys

J.S. Baker[1], A. Leyshon[2], M.G. Hughes[2], B. Davies[3], M. Graham[4], and N.E. Thomas[5]

[1]University of the West of Scotland, UK; [2]University of Wales Institute Cardiff, UK; [3]University of Glamorgan, UK; [4]Newman University College, UK; [5]Swansea University, UK

18.1   INTRODUCTION

For the most part, children and adolescents' physical activity (PA) patterns involve short bursts of dynamic activities interspersed with periods of recovery (Baquet *et al.*, 2007). These PA bouts might occur during regular physical education (PE) lessons, organized sports practice, or free play. Despite frequently engaging in brief bouts of high-intensity exercise, there is a dearth of information available on the physiological response of children and adolescents to this type of activity (Armstrong *et al.*, 2001). Specifically, there appear to be few data examining the response of stress hormones and immunological parameters to repeated, high-intensity exercise in this age group.

We investigated the effect of repeated bouts of short-term, high-intensity cycling exercise on the salivary cortisol, testosterone and immunoglobulin (A) concentrations of 15-16 year old boys.

18.2   METHODS

Seventeen apparently healthy schoolchildren (aged 15.5 ± 0.4 years) participated in this study. Written parental consent and participants' assent were obtained prior to the study. A health questionnaire was completed by the parents confirming that the participants had not recently suffered from an upper respiratory tract illness including sore throat, runny nose, headache, or fever. The schoolchildren were habituated to the laboratory environment and experimental procedures. All experimental procedures were carried out over two mornings, at least three hours after a light breakfast. The participants were instructed not to engage in strenuous activity during the day before an exercise test. The study was given approval by the University's ethics committee.

18.2.1 Anthropometric measurements

Stature was measured using a portable stadiometer (Holtain Ltd, Crymych, Pembrokeshire, UK). Body mass (BM) was recorded using a Phillips electronic scale (HP 5320). Skinfold measurements were taken with Harpenden skinfold calipers (John Bull, British Indicators Ltd, Bedfordshire, UK). The protocol was performed in triplicate; and triceps and subscapular thicknesses were used to estimate percent body fat (%BF). Fat free mass (FFM) was calculated using the equation BM – (%BF x BM/100). For maturation status, the participants were given a gender-specific questionnaire and asked to complete this in private.

All participants completed 6 x 8 secs sprints, interspersed with 30 secs recovery intervals on a cycle ergometer. Participants were harnessed to the ergometer so that they remained seated during the exercise. Toe clips were used to prevent the feet from slipping off the pedals. Prior to the test, all participants completed a standardised warm-up which consisted of three minutes pedalling against 0.5kg at 60rpm, interspersed with two maximal effort sprints of 2-3 seconds. The resistive force of 0.075kg·kg-1 (0.74N·kg-1) was used throughout. The participants were given a rolling start at 60rpm for a 5 second period against minimal resistance. On the command "3-2-1-go!" the participants commenced maximal effort pedalling and the resistive force applied simultaneously. Each participant was given verbal encouragement to perform maximally for each sprint. Immediately post–test, all participants completed a cool down consisting of continuous light pedalling at 30W for three minutes.

The following indices of high intensity performance were recorded: peak power output (PPO) (watts); mean power output (MPO) (watts); and fatigue index (FI) (%). Heart rate was measured pre, during, and post exercise (up to 5 min) using short-range telemetry (Sports Tester 3000, Polar Electro Finland).

18.2.2 Saliva measurements

The participants provided unstimulated saliva samples at rest, and five minutes post exercise. Saliva samples were collected by participants using the passive drool method. Salivary measures of cortisol and testosterone were determined by expanded range enzyme immunoassay (Salimetrics, State College, PA 16803 USA). The intra and inter assay variations for cortisol were: intra: 3.5-3.65%; inter: 3.75-6.41%. The intra and inter assay variations for testosterone were: intra: 2.5-6.7%; inter: 7.9-8.6%. Salivary Ig(A) was determined using an in-house quantitative enzyme linked immunosorbent assay (ELISA) protocol. The intra and inter assay variations were less than 10%.

18.2.3 Statistical analysis

The experimental values are expressed as mean ± standard deviation (mean ± SD). A Student's t-test was used to identify differences between SalC, SalT and SIgA, pre and post exercise. The threshold for statistical significance was set at $p = 0.05$.

18.3   RESULTS

Age and anthropometric data are presented in Table 18.1. Power indices for the group are presented in Table 18.2. Best PPO values (i.e., participants' best PPO from six sprints) for this cohort ranged from 530.9 to 1326.7 watts. All the boys reported stages of 4 or 5 for pubic hair and genitalia development. A comparison of pre and post exercise SalC, SalT and SIgA is included in Table 18.3. There were significant changes ($p \leq 0.05$) in both SalT and SalC, five mins after high intensity exercise. No significant differences ($p > 0.05$) were recorded for SIg(A).

Table 18.1. Mean ± SD for age and anthropometric values.

	Mean ± SD ($n = 17$)
Age (yr)	15.5 ± 0.4
Stature (cm)	164.7± 8.1
Body mass (kg)	59.1± 12.6
BF (%)	22.8 ± 7.9
FFM (kg)	44.8 ± 6.1

BF: body fat; FFM: fat free mass.

Table 18.2. Power indices and heart rates.

Variable	Mean ± SD ($n = 17$)
PPO (watts)	723.1 ± 180.3
Max FI%	43.3 ± 8.3
APPO (watts)	605.9 ± 81.7
AMPO (watts)	483.6 ± 68.1
HR pre (beats/min)	85.7 ± 10.8
HR post (beats/min)	176.1 ± 26.9

PPO: peak power output (best PPO from 6 sprints); Max FI%: Greatest fatigue index value; APPO: average peak power output (across 6 sprints); AMPO: average mean power output (across 6 sprints); HR: heart rate.

Table 18.3. Concentrations (mean ± SD) of SalC, SalT and SIgA at pre, and 5 min post, 6 x 8 s sprints with 30 s recovery ($n = 17$).

	SalC (ug/dl)	SalT (pg/ml)	SIg(A) (ng/ml)
Pre exercise	0.13± 0.69	66.19 ± 23.18	520 ± 499
Post exercise	0.20 ± 0.12*	88.03 ± 33.78*	482.5 ± 203.9

*denotes significance ($p \leq 0.05$) difference between pre and post exercise.

18.4   CONCLUSION

Children and adolescents playing in uninhibited conditions naturally engage in brief bouts of high-intensity exercise; therefore, an enhanced understanding of their hormonal and immunological responses to maximal exercise would be helpful.

Concurring with previous research salivary testosterone increased ($p \leq 0.05$) following exercise (Viru *et al.*, 1999; Di Luigi *et al.*, 2006). Post exercise cortisone concentrations were similarly elevated ($p \leq 0.05$), a finding that it is in agreement with some (Di Luigi *et al.*, 2006), but not all research evidence (Hershberger *et al.*, 2004). Exercise would normally be expected to increase cortisol level; however, the changes are not immediately evident on cessation of activity. According to Lac *et al.* (1999), the rise in cortisol level will appear only after a minimal delay of 20 min; hence, there is a possibility that a later post exercise measurement in our study might have produced yet higher hormonal responses. There are few data relating to young people that have examined the influence of repeated maximal exercise on the immune system. Although our study reported a decrease in SIg(A) concentration following short-term, high-intensity exercise, this was not significant ($p > 0.05$). This suggests that a threshold intensity and/or duration must be achieved if a hormonal response is to occur in 15–16 year old boys (Viru *et al.*, 1996).

The findings presented here contribute to existing research in relation to the measured hormonal and immune function responses to high-intensity repeat exercise in 15–16 year old boys.

18.5   REFERENCES

Armstrong, N., Welsman, J.R. and Chia, M.Y.H., 2001, Short term power output in relation to growth and maturation. *British Journal of Sports Medicine*, **35**, p. 118–124.

Baquet, G., Stratton, G., Van Praagh, E. and Berthoin, S., 2007, Improving physical   activity assessment in prepubertal children with high-frequency accelerometry monitoring: a methodological issue. *Preventive Medicine*, **44**, pp. 143–147

Di Luigi, L., Baldari, C., Gallotta, M.C., Perroni, F., Romanelli, F., Lenzi, A. and Guidetti, L., 2006, Salivary steroids at rest and after a training load in young male athletes: relationship with chronological age and pubertal development. *International Journal of Sports Medicine*, **27**, pp. 709–717.

Hershberger, A.M., McCammon, M.R., Harry, J.P., Mahar, M.T. and Hickner, R.C., 2004, Responses of lipolysis and salivary cortisol to food intake and physical activity in lean and obese children. *Journal of Clinical Endocrinology and Metabolism*, **89**, pp. 4701–4707.

Lac, G., Marquet, P., Chassaing, A.P. and Galen, F.X., 1999, Dexamethasone in resting and exercising men: Effects on adrenocorticol hormones. *Journal of Applied Physiology*, **87**, pp. 183–188.

Viru, A., Smirnova, T., Karelson, K., Snegovskaya, V. and Viru, M., 1996, Determinants and modulators of hormonal responses to exercise. *Biology of Sport*, **13**, pp. 169–187.

Viru, A., Viru, M. and Kuusler, K., 1999, Exercise-induced hormonal response in boys in relation to sexual maturation. In: XXth International Symposium of the European Group of Pediatric Work Physiology, pp. 135.

Part IV

Cardiorespiratory Functions

HCO$_3^-$ and non-Respiratory HCO$_3^-$ Buffering in Boys and Male Adolescents

R. Beneke[1], M. Hütler[2], and R.M. Leithäuser[1]

[1]University of Essex, UK; [2]Haukeland Universityhospital, Bergen, Norway

19.1 INTRODUCTION

The respiratory response to exercise seems to be faster at younger age resulting in lower carbon dioxide partial pressure (pCO_2) at given pH and bicarbonate concentrations (HCO$_3^-$) in children than in adults (Hebestreit *et al.* 1996; Ratel *et al.*, 2002). The relationship between changes in plasma HCO$_3^-$ and pH can serve as a quantitative measure of the extra-cellular HCO$_3^-$ related pH defense (ß_{HCO}). It reflects a buffer capacity determined by titration in plasma under in vivo and in vitro conditions including respiratory compensation (RESPC) related decreases of pCO_2 (Parkhouse and McKenzie, 1984; Siggaard-Andersen, 1974; Sahlin, 1978; Böning, 1974).

We tested the hypotheses a) that pH defense is faster, b) that pCO_2 control is tighter and c) that the smaller decrease in pH combined with tighter pCO_2 control, lower pCO_2 at given pH and HCO$_3^-$ reflect a lower $\text{ß}_{HCO\_non\text{-}RESPC}$ in boys than in male adolescents.

19.2 METHODS

19.2.1 Subjects and procedures

Eight pre- or early pubescent boys and eight late or post pubertal male adolescents (age: 11.7 ± 0.3 vs. 16.5 ± 0.7 yrs, height: 151.0 ± 5.9 vs. 184 ± 7.2 cm, body mass: 39.1 ± 3.9 vs. 70.5 ± 8.0 kg, all $p < 0.001$) participated in the present study and performed a 30 s Wingate Anaerobic Test (WAnT) on a mechanically braked cycle ergometer (834 E, Monark). Capillary blood samples were drawn from the hyperaemic ear lobe. 85 µl were taken immediately before and at 1, 5, 10, 15 and 20 min after the test for pH, pCO_2 and HCO$_3^-$ analyses (ABL510, Radiometer).

19.2.2 Data processing

The dynamics of the pH response to every individual WAnT was analyzed using a 3-parameter bi-exponential model (Beneke *et al.*, 2005). Additionally the relative change in pH as related to the highest decrease measured during WAnT-recovery was calculated.

HCO_3^- buffering was calculated as change in HCO_3^- ($DHCO_3^-$) over the corresponding change in pH (DpH), and the non-respiratory component of HCO_3^- buffering by calculation of HCO_3^- for a constant pCO_2 of 40 mmHg and relating the resulting $DHCO_3^-_{non-RESPC}$ to the corresponding DpH. The capacity of $DHCO_3^-$ ($ß_{HCO}$) and $DHCO_3^-_{non-RESPC}$ ($ß_{HCO\_non-RESPC}$) was calculated as individual regression coefficients of the reciprocal slope of DpH over $DHCO_3^-$ and $DHCO_3^-_{non-RESPC}$ since $DHCO_3^-$ and $DHCO_3^-_{non-RESPC}$ are physiologically the independent variable.

19.2.3 Statistics

Descriptive results are reported as mean values and standard deviations (SD). The general interrelationships between $DHCO_3^-$ and DpH and $DHCO_3^-_{non-RESPC}$ and $DpH_{non-RESPC}$ were tested by non-linear regression. Differences in performance between boys and adolescents were tested using independent t-test. Effects of age and recovery on acid base control were tested using an age group x sample time ANOVA model with tukey and independent t-tests as post hoc analyses. For all statistics, the significance level was set at $p < 0.05$.

19.3   RESULTS

In boys pH was higher ($p < 0.05$) than in adolescents in all post WAnT samples. In spite of the lower amplitude of the pH response in the boys compared to the adolescents no difference in the rate constants of pH increase (0.96 ± 0.17 vs. 0.75 ± 0.27 min^{-1}) and decrease (0.06 ± 0.01 vs. 0.05 ± 0.1 min^{-1}) of the time of the pH-minimum were found (Figure 19.1).

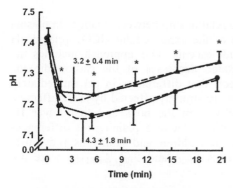
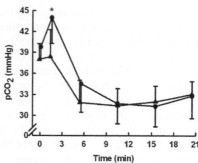

Figure 19.1 pH does not recover to pre test values in boys (▲) and in adolescents (●) during 20 min of passive recovery; measured pH (solid lines), modeled pH (dotted lines); *: different between boy and adolescents.

Figure 19.2. pCO₂ does not recover to pre test values in boys (▲) and in adolescents (●) during 20 min of passive recovery; *: different between boy and adolescents.

Also the relative changes in pH during WAnT-recovery were not different between boys and adolescents. pCO_2 was lower ($p < 0.05$) in boys than in adolescents 1 min post WAnT (Figure 19.2).

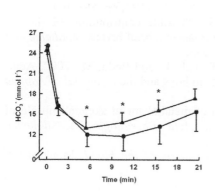
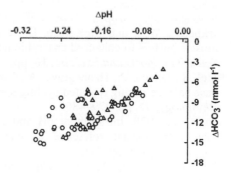

Figure 19.3. HCO₃⁻ in boys (▲) and in adolescents (●) do not recover to pre test values during 20 min of passive recovery; *: different between boy and adolescents.

Figure 19.4. Interrelationship between DHCO₃⁻ and DpH in boys (△) and adolescents (○) (all data pooled).

HCO_3^- was higher ($p < 0.05$) in boys than in adolescents at min 5, 10 and 15 min post WAnT (Figure 19.3). The interrelationship between DHCO₃⁻ and DpH (Figure 19.4), ß$_{HCO}$ (62.3 ± 5.0 vs. 59.8 ± 6.1 mmol l⁻¹) and ß$_{HCO\_non-RESPC}$ (47.7 ± 2.5 vs. 45.7 ± 3.2 mmol l⁻¹) were not different between boys and adolescents.

19.4   CONCLUSIONS

The present study is the first analyzing the relationship between changes in plasma HCO_3^- and pH as a quantitative measure of the extra-cellular HCO_3^- related pH defense post WAnT in boys and male adolescents. This approach includes the $HCO_3^-{}_{non\text{-}RESPC}$–buffering and RESPC related decreases of the carbon dioxide partial pressure. The present results support that differences in pH immediately post WAnT between boys and adolescents are strongly affected by more effective RESPC during and immediately post WAnT in the boys and that lower H^+ concentrations in the boys serve as an additional factor explaining the differences in HCO_3^- and H^+ to pCO_2 ratios between children and adults as previously described (Ratel *et al.*, 2002). Nevertheless ß$_{HCO}$ and ß$_{HCO\_non\text{-}RESPC}$ were not different between boys and adolescents.

19.5   REFERENCES

Beneke, R., Hütler, M., Jung, M. and Leithäuser, R.M., 2005, Modeling the blood lactate kinetics at maximal short-term exercise conditions in children, adolescents and adults. *Journal of Applied Physiology*, **99**, pp. 499-504.

Böning, D., 1974, The "in vivo" and "in vitro" CO_2-equilibration curves of blood during acute hypercapnia and hypocapnia. II. Theoretical considerations. *Pflügers Archive*, **350**, pp. 213–222.

Hebestreit, H., Meyer, F., Heigenhauser, G.J. and Bar-Or, O., 1996, Plasma metabolites, volume and electrolytes following 30-s high-intensity exercise in boys and men. *European Journal of Applied Physiology*, **72**, pp. 563-569.

Parkhouse, W.S. and McKenzie, D.C., 1984, Possible contributions of skeletal muscle buffers to enhanced anaerobic performance: a brief review. *Medicine and Science in Sports and Exercise*, **16**, pp. 328-338.

Ratel, S., Duche, P., Hennegrave, A., Van Praagh, E. and Bedu, M., 2002, Acid-base balance during repeated cycling sprints in boys and men. *Journal of Applied Physiology*, **92**, pp. 479–485.

Sahlin, K., 1978, Intracellular pH and energy metabolism in skeletal muscle of men with special reference to exercise. *Acta Physiologica Scandinavica Supplement*, **455**, pp. 1-56.

Siggaard-Andersen, O., 1974, *The acid–base status of the blood.* Munksgaard, Copenhagen.

Secular Trends in Established and Emerging Cardiovascular Risk Factors in Welsh Adolescents

N.E. Thomas[1], R. Williams[1], D.A. Rowe[2], B. Davies[3], and J.S. Baker[4]

[1] Swansea University, UK; [2] University of Strathclyde, UK; [3] University of Glamorgan, UK; [4] University of the West of Scotland, UK

20.1   INTRODUCTION

Cardiovascular disease (CVD) continues to be the leading cause of death in developed countries (British Heart Foundation, 2003). Research evidence indicates that many of the precursors of CVD originate in childhood, and that they progress through the life span. Importantly, these risk factors are preventable: their development at an early age is closely related to health behaviour, particularly inactive lifestyles and lipid-rich diets (Raitakuri et al., 2003).

The primary prevention of CVD should begin early in childhood, with appropriate healthy lifestyle patterns established. Any changes in the prevalence of CVD risk factors among specific populations should be reflected in the design and implementation of lifestyle interventions. Examining secular trends provides us with an important insight into the seemingly upward trend in overweight and obesity, as well as other CVD risk factors. There is a dearth of information on the secular trends of CVD risk factors in British adolescents; there are none for young people living in Wales. Our study presents a current and comprehensive examination of secular trends in established and emerging CVD risk factors among Welsh 12-13 year olds from 2002 to 2007.

20.2   METHODS

We examined CVD risk factor data from two cross-sectional studies. The first study (73 participants; aged 12.9 ± 0.3 years) was completed during Sept-Oct, 2002. The second study (90 participants; aged 12.9 ± 0.4 years) was conducted from Sept-Oct, 2007. Letters of information and consent forms were distributed to the parents of all participants. All participants were assured of anonymity and informed that they were free to withdraw from the project at any time. On both occasions, free school meal eligibility was used as a measure of socio-economic status (Shuttleworth, 1995). The study's protocol was approved by the University's Ethics Committee.

Measurements included body mass index (BMI), waist circumference (WC), physical activity (PA), physical fitness (PF), diet, total cholesterol (TC), high-density-lipoprotein cholesterol (HDL-C), low-density-lipoprotein cholesterol (LDL-C), triglyceride (TG), fibrinogen (Fg), and high-sensitivity C-reactive protein (hs-CRP). Blood samples were collected between 9am and 10.30am, and following an overnight fast. To control for plasma volume shifts, venous blood was sampled after the participants had assumed a seated position for at least 30 minutes (Pronk, 1993). Blood samples were allowed to clot and then centrifuged at 3,500 rpm for 10 min. Total cholesterol and TG concentrations were estimated by routine enzymatic techniques using the Vitros 950 System (Ortho-Clinical Diagnostics, Amersham, Bucks). The concentration of HDL-C was determined after precipitation of very low-density and low-density lipoproteins with dextran sulphate and magnesium chloride. Low density lipoprotein-cholesterol concentration was calculated by the Friedewald formula (Friedewald *et al.*, 1972). Fibrinogen concentration was determined according to the method of Clauss and using the ACL Futura Analyzer (Instrumentation Laboratory Company, Lexington, MA) (Clauss, 1957). C-reactive protein concentration was measured by an immunoturbidimetric method using the Cobas Fara (Roche, Welwyn Garden, UK). Coefficients of variance for the laboratory measures of TC, HDL-C, TG, Fg, and hs-CRP were 1.6%, 5.3%, 2%, 1.6%, and 5.5%, respectively.

An independent group t-test was used to identify whether differences in the means for CVD risk factors existed between 2002 and 2007 cohorts. To improve the distribution of this variable, CRP levels were logarithmically transformed in all analyses. The level of significance set at $p < .05$.

20.3 RESULTS

The descriptive statistics for boys and girls are summarised in Tables 20.1 and 20.2, respectively. Parametric data are also presented in Tables 20.1 and 20.2. In boys only, mean BMI and WC decreased between 2002 and 2007, but this was not significant ($p \geq .05$) (Table 20.1). Generally, there were significant improvements in mean lipid profile, Fg and hs-CRP ($p < .05$) (Tables 20.1 and 20.2). In 2002, 42.8 per cent of boys, and 34.2 per cent of girls, were overweight or obese; in 2007, this was 23.7 per cent and 28.9 per cent for boys and girls, respectively. More adolescents in the earlier cohort exceeded the recommended levels for lipids. This was also true for Fg and hs-CRP (Table 20.3). The response rates were: 88% in 2002; 80% in 2007.

Table 20.1. Cross-sectional secular trends (mean ± SD) for established and emerging CVD risk factors in Welsh 12-13 year old boys.

	2002 n =35	2007 n =38	p
Age (yrs)	12.9 ± 0.3	12.9 ± 0.6	
BMI (kg/m^2)	21.5 ± 3.8	20.3 ± 3.6	.19
WC (cm)	70.1 ± 10.4	67.8 ± 8.9	.32
TC (mmol/L)	4.18 ± 0.73	3.81 ± 0.68	.03*
HDL-C (mmol/L)	1.34 ± 0.32	1.62 ± 0.35	.00*
LDL-C (mmol/L)	2.4 ± 0.62	1.90 ± 0.57	.00*
TC:HDL-C	3.27 ± 0.91	2.42 ± 0.53	.00*
TG (mmol/L)	0.98 ± 0.46	0.61 ± 0.28	.00*
Fg (g/L)	4.42 ± 0.99	2.74 ± 0.4	.00*
hs-CRP (mg/L)	1.50 ± 1.52	0.63 ± 0.73	.01*

BMI = body mass index; WC = waist circumference; TC = total cholesterol; HDL-C = high-density lipoprotein; LDL-C low-density lipoprotein; TC:HDL-C = ratio total cholesterol to high-density lipoprotein; TG = triglyceride; Fg = fibrinogen; hs-CRP = high-sensitivity C-reactive protein.

Table 20.2. Cross-sectional secular trends (mean ± SD) for established and emerging CVD risk factors in Welsh 12-13 year old girls.

	2002 n =38	2007 n −52	p
Age (yrs)	12.9 ± 0.3	12.9 ± 0.5	
BMI (kg/m^2)	21.2 ± 3.1	21.1 ± 3.5	.97
WC (cm)	63.7 ± 7.6	65.7 ± 7.9	.25
TC (mmol/L)	4.39 ± 0.59	4.11 + 0.64	.04*
HDL-C (mmol/L)	1.44 ± 0.32	1.69 + 0.33	.00*
LDL-C (mmol/L)	2.5 ± 0.49	2.09 ± 0.55	.00*
TC:HDL-C	3.18 ± 0.72	2.5 ± 0.47	.00*
TG (mmol/L)	1 ± 0.48	0.79 ± 0.31	.02*
Fg (g/L)	3.9 ± 0.83	2.7 ± 0.5	.00*
hs-CRP (mg/L)	1.57 ± 2.07	0.36 ± 0.54	.00*

BMI = body mass index; WC = waist circumference; TC = total cholesterol; HDL-C = high-density lipoprotein; LDL-C low-density lipoprotein; TC:HDL-C = ratio total cholesterol to high-density lipoprotein; TG = triglyceride; Fg = fibrinogen; hs-CRP = high-sensitivity C-reactive protein.

Table 20.3. Percentage of participants exceeding thresholds in 2002 and 2007.

Boys	2002 (n =35)	2007 (n =38)	Girls	2002 (n =38)	2007 (n =52)
BMI			BMI		
Overweight	37.1%	15.8%	overweight	34.2%	23.1%
Obese	5.7%	7.9%	Obese	0%	5.8%
TC	11.8%	3.0%	TC	7.9%	3.7%
HDL-C	11.8%	0%	HDL-C	7.9%	0%
LDL-C	0%	0%	LDL-C	0%	1.9%
TC:HDL-C	23.5%	0%	TC:HDL-C	18.4%	0%
TG	8.8%	0%	TG	3.0%	1.9%
Fg	73.5%	3.0%	Fg	63.2%	18.4%
hs-CRP	8.8%	3.0%	hs-CRP	18.4%	1.9%

BMI = body mass index; WC = waist circumference; TC = total cholesterol; HDL-C = high-density lipoprotein; LDL-C low-density lipoprotein; TC:HDL-C = ratio total cholesterol to high-density lipoprotein; TG = triglyceride; Fg = fibrinogen; hs-CRP = high-sensitivity C-reactive protein.

20.4   CONCLUSION

To our knowledge, and despite CVD having its genesis in young people, this is the only study to examine established and emerging CVD risk factor trends in Welsh schoolchildren. In this study, a range of CVD risk factor measures was undertaken in the same school, five years apart (in 2002 and 2007). All anthropometric and physiological measures were performed by the same experienced researcher, using identical methodologies, at the same time of year, and on the same age group. All blood samples underwent the same storage and assay procedures. The social make-up of pupil intake at the school, as depicted by free school meal status, did not change significantly between 2002 and 2007.

Despite our finding that overweight is widespread in Welsh adolescents, we did not identify an increased prevalence in our later cohort. Moreover, our findings present a positive trend in lipid profile during the five year time span. In an earlier publication, we reported significant improvements in physical activity (PA) and physical fitness (PF), but no change in dietary habits or mean adiposity measures between 2002 and 2007 (Thomas *et al.* in press). Although there is insufficient evidence to conclude that superior fitness improves lipid status in adolescents (Thomas *et al.*, 2003), it is possible that, in our 2007 cohort, higher PA and PF may have contributed to the enhanced lipid profile.

There is little information on secular trends in emerging CVD risk factors among adolescents. In our cohorts, we measured two inflammatory factors, namely, Fg and hs-CRP. Significant improvements were reported in Fg and hs-CRP levels between 2002 and 2007; this was true for boys and girls. Since this improvement corresponds with an enhanced lipid status, it is possible that the health of schoolchildren at this school has improved over five years. However, although Fg and hs-CRP are independent risk factors for CVD, they are also acute phase proteins, hence any elevated concentrations in the 2002 cohort might have been in response to an acute infection. Although participants were requested to report any recent episodes of acute illnesses or infections, it is feasible that they were unaware of their presence.

In conclusion, the current worldwide epidemic of childhood obesity has led to extensive efforts in prevention. More studies are urgently needed to confirm our findings, and any changes in the prevalence of CVD risk factors among specific populations should be reflected in the design of future preventive measures.

20.5 REFERENCES

British Heart Foundation, 2003, Coronary heart disease statistics. Available at: www.dphpcox.ac.uk/bhfhprg/stats.

Clauss, A., 1957, Schnellmethode zur Bestimmung des Fibrinogens. *Acta Haematolgica*, **17**, pp. 237–247.

Friedewald, W.T., Levy, I. and Fredrickson, D.S., 1972, Estimation of the Concentration of low-density lipoprotein cholesterol in plasma, without the use of the preparative centrifuge'. *Clinical Chemistry*, **18**, pp. 499–502.

Pronk, N.P., 1993, Short term effects of exercise on plasma lipids and lipoproteins in humans. *Sports Medicine*, **16**, pp. 431–448.

Raitakari, O.T., Juonala, M., Kahonen, M., Taittonen, L., Laitinen, T., Mäki-Torkko, N., Järvisalo, M.J., Uhari, M., Jokinen, E., Rönnemaa, T., Åkerblom, H.K. and Viikari, J.S.A., 2003, Cardiovascular risk factors in childhood and carotid artery intima-media thickness in adulthood. *Journal of the American Medical Association*, **90**, pp. 2277–2283.

Shuttleworth, I., 1995, The relationship between social deprivation as measured by individual free school meal eligibility and educational attainment at GCSE in Northern Ireland: a preliminary investigation. *British Educational Research Journal*, **21**, pp. 487–504.

Thomas, N.E., Baker, J.S. and Davies, B., 2003, Established and recently identified coronary heart disease risk factors in young people and the influence of physical activity and physical fitness on these risk factors. *Sports Medicine*, **33**, pp. 633–650.

Thomas, N.E., Baker, J.S., Rowe, D., Davies, B. and Baker, J.S, A time-related study of cardiovascular disease risk factors in a similar socio-economic status cohort of schoolchildren. *Health Educational Journal* (in press).

Limiting Factors in Maximum Oxygen Uptake in Ambulatory Children with Spina Bifida

J.F. De Groot[1,2], T. Takken[2], M.A.G.C. Schoenmakers[2],
L. Vanhees[1,3], and P.J.M. Helders[2]

[1]Research Group Lifestyle and Health, University of Applied Sciences, Utrecht,
The Netherlands; [2]Child Development & Exercise Center, Wilhelmina Children's
Hospital, University Medical Center Utrecht, the Netherlands; [3]Department of
Rehabilitation Sciences, Catholic University Leuven, Leuven, Belgium

21.1 INTRODUCTION

Earlier studies have shown children and young adults with SB to be less active with reduced levels of physical fitness compared to their healthy peers (Steele *et al.*, 1996; van den Berg-Emons *et al.*, 2003; Agre *et al.*, 1987). Based on these results, Van den Berg-Emons *et al.* (2003) concluded that programs aimed at regular physical exercise and daily physical activity should be started in childhood to prevent further decline in physical fitness and daily functioning. In our SB clinic 23 ambulatory children with SB were seen for sports and lifestyle advice. Results showed low levels of overall muscle strength, exercise capacity and daily physical activity (Schoenmakers *et al.*, 2009). While designing an exercise program aimed at improving both endurance and ambulation in ambulatory children with SB, the question was raised which factors in terms of cardiovascular, pulmonary or muscular were limiting $\dot{V}O_{2peak}$ in these children (De Groot *et al.*, 2008). In this pilot study, we found signs for both deconditioning and -much to our surprise-possible signs of insufficient gas exchange at the pulmonary level as indicated by high ventilatory equivalents for CO_2 uptake. We then concluded future exercise testing in ambulatory children with SB should include evaluation of the ventilatory reserve and desaturation to better determine possible ventilatory limitations. The aim of this study was again to look at the limiting factors in exercise testing, but using additional measurements to evaluate the ventilatory limitations.

21.2   METHODS

A cross-sectional study, in Wilhelmina's Children's Hospital Utrecht, the Netherlands, including 49 ambulatory children (age: 10.7 ± 3 years) with SB.

Peak oxygen uptake ($\dot{V}O_{2peak}$) was measured during a graded treadmill-test. In order to accommodate children with different ambulatory abilities, two progressive exercise test protocols were used. Children ambulating <400 meters during a six-minute walking test (6MWT), were tested with a starting speed of 2 km/h, which was gradually increased by 0.25 km/h every minute, with a set grade of 2%. Children ambulating >400 meters during the 6MWT, were started at a speed of 3 km/h, with the speed being increased 0.50 km/h every minute, with a set grade of 2% (De Groot *et al.*, 2009). Prior to exercise testing, FEV_1 was determined using incentive spirometry to calculate maximum voluntary ventilation ($40 \times FEV_1$).

Eschenbacher's and Maninna's algorithm (Eschenbacher and Mannina, 1990) was used to determine limiting factors for $\dot{V}O_{2peak}$. Ventilatory reserve (VR) $\leq$ 30% of maximum ventilatory volume, ventilatory coefficients for exhaled carbon dioxide ($\dot{V}_E/\dot{V}CO_2$) $\geq$ 35 and oxygen desaturation of $\geq$ 4% were evaluated for possible ventilatory limitations. Heart rate response (HRR) $\geq$ predicted for age and % $\dot{V}O_2$ at Anaerobic Threshold (AT) $\leq$ 40% of $\dot{V}O_{2peak}$ were evaluated for possible cardiac limitations and deconditioning. Cut-off points were adapted for the pediatric population.

Descriptive statistics were used. Statistical analyses were performed using SPSS for Windows (version 15.0, SPSS Inc, Chicago, Ill.).

21.3   RESULTS

$\dot{V}O_{2peak}$ was significantly lower compared to reference values. $\dot{V}O_{2peak}$, HR_{peak}, RER_{peak} can be found in Table 21.1. Outcomes of the algorithm can be found in Table 21.2. Looking at the ventilatory limitations, VR was low in 54%, $\dot{V}_E/\dot{V}CO_2$ was high in 60%, while 6% of the children showed desaturation $\geq$ 4% during exercise, indicating ventilatory mechanical limitations in exercise testing. HRR was high in 55%. AT was reached in 82.7% and was $\geq$ 40% in most (98%) children, indicating deconditioning and/or muscular components rather than circulatory limitations in low $\dot{V}O_{2peak}$.

Table 21.1. Outcomes of maximal exercise testing.

Outcomes of Maximal Exercise Testing	Value
$\dot{V}O_{2peak}$ (ml/min/kg)	34.4 (8.8)
Z-scores	-2.55 (1.6)
HR_{peak} (beats/min)	180 (23)
RER_{peak}	0.99 (0.1)
AT reached	82.4 %

$\dot{V}O_{2peak}$: peak oxygen uptake; HR_{peak}: peak heart rate; RER_{peak}: peak respiratory exchange ratio, AT: anaerobic threshold.

Table 21.2. Percentages reaching critical values in algorithm of Eschenbacher and Maninna (1990).

Parameter*	% reaching cut off values	Indicative for…
Ventilatory Reserve < 30%	54 %	Ventilatory mechanical limitations
Ventilatory Coefficient for $\dot{V}CO_2 > 35$	60 %	Gas exchange abnormalities
Oxygen desaturation > 4%	6 %	Diffusion limitations
Heart Rate Response > (-6.25 × age) + 150	55 %	Deconditioning/cardiac myopathy
$\dot{V}O_2$ at Anaerobic Threshold < 40%	2 %	Deconditioning/poor cardiac pump function

* adapted to pediatric values based on data from a sample of 50 healthy Dutch children.

21.4   CONCLUSION

The aim of this study was to look more closely at the limiting factors during maximum exercise testing in ambulatory children with SB. $\dot{V}O_{2peak}$ in ambulatory children seems to be limited by both ventilatory mechanical limitations and "deconditioning and/or muscular" limitations. The use of additional parameters to determine ventilatory limitations, had resulted in an increase of these limitations. Where the latter can be explained by both the disease and reduced physical activity level, the ventilatory limitations need further investigation. In the literature, one other article reports on pulmonary dysfunction in spina bifida (Shermans *et al.*, 1997). Hypothetical causes for ventilatory limitations include abnormal control of ventilation, short trachea, kyphoscoliosis and reduced inspiratory muscle strength due to deconditioning. Another possible explanation of these high ventilatory equivalents might be the presence of a Chiari II malformation, often present in children with SB. This malformation affects the brain stem and is known to influence ventilation and O_2 and CO_2 peripheral chemoreceptor function in children with SB (Gozal *et al.*, 1995; Petersen *et al.*, 1995). In the meantime, exercise training seems indicated to reverse the effects of deconditioning in ambulatory children with SB.

21.5 REFERENCES

Agre, J.C., Findley, T.W., McNally, M.C., Habeck, R., Leon, A.S., Stradel, L., Birkebak, R. and Schmalz, R., 1987, Physical activity capacity in children with myelomeningocele. *Archives of Physical Medicine and Rehabilitation*, **68**, pp. 372–377.

De Groot, J.F., Takken, T., de Graaff, S., Gooskens, R.H., Helders, P.J.M. and Vanhees, L., 2009, Treadmill testing of children who have spina bifida and are ambulatory: does peak oxygen uptake reflect maximum oxygen uptake? *Physical Therapy*, **89**, pp. 679–687.

De Groot, J.F., Takken, T., Schoenmakers, M.A.C.G., Vanhees, L. and Helders, P.J.M., 2008, Interpretation of maximal exercise testing and the relationship with ambulation parameters in ambulation children with Spina Bifida. *European Journal of Applied Physiology,* **104**, pp. 657–665.

Eschenbacher, W.L. and Mannina, A., 1990, An algoritm for the interpretation of cardiopulmonary exercise tests. *Chest,* **97**, pp. 263–267.

Gozal., D, Arens, R., Omlin, K.J., Jacobs, R.A. and Keens, T.G., 1995, Peripheral chemoreceptor function in children with myelomeningocele and Arnold-Chiari malformation type 2. *Chest*, **108**, pp. 425–431.

Petersen, M.C., Wolraich, M., Sherbondy, A. and Wagener, J., 1995, Abnormalities in control of ventilation in newborn infants with myelomeningocele. *Journal of Pediatrics*, **126**, pp. 1011–1015.

Schoenmakers, M.A.G.C., De Groot, J.F., Gorter, J.W., Hilleart, J.L.M., Helders, P.J.M. and Takken, T., 2009, Muscle strength, aerobic capacity and physical activity in independent ambulating children with lumbosacral spina bifida. *Disability and Rehabilitation*, **31**, pp. 259–266.

Shermans, M.S., Kaplan, J.M., Effgen, S., Campbell, D. and Dold, F., 1997, Pulmonary dysfunction and reduced exercise capacity in patients with myelomeningocele. *Journal of Pediatrics*, **131**, pp. 413–418.

Steele, C.A., Kalnins, I.V., Jutai, J.W., Stevens, S.E., Bortolussi, J.A. and Biggar, W.D., 1996, Lifestyle health behaviours of 11-16 year old youth with physical disabilities. *Health and Education Research,* **11**, pp. 173–186.

van den Berg-Emons, H.J., Bussmann, J.B., Meyerink, H.J., Roebroeck, M.E. and Stam, H.J., 2003, Body fat, fitness and level of everyday physical activity in adolescents and young adults with meningomyelocele. *Journal of Rehabilitation Medicine,* **35**, pp. 271–275.

Cardiopulmonary Exercise Test Characteristics of Children with End-Stage Renal Disease: Signs of an Acquired Myopathy?

T. Takken[1], R. Engelbert[1], M. van Bergen[1], J. Groothoff[2], J. Nauta[3], K. van Hoeck[4], M. Lilien[1], and P.J.M. Helders[1]

[1]Wilhelmina Children's Hospital, Utrecht; [2]Emma Children's Hospital, Amsterdam; [3]Sophia Children's Hospital, Rotterdam, the Netherlands; [4]University Hospital Antwerp, Antwerp, Belgium

22.1 INTRODUCTION

Children with end-stage renal disease (ESRD) are characterized by multiple factors that influence their exercise capacity like anaemia, metabolic acidosis, electrolyte imbalance, osteopenia, growth failure, malnutrition, fluid imbalance, muscle wasting and a sedentary life style (Bar-Or and Rowland, 2004, Painter *et al.*, 2007). Increased exercise capacity ($\dot{V}O_{2peak}$) was reported in adult and pediatric dialysis patients after treatment for anemia using erythropoietin (Robertson *et al.*, 1990; Warady *et al.*, 1991), although the $\dot{V}O_{2peak}$ response to increasing hematocrit in patients on dialysis was clearly blunted compared with healthy subjects (Painter, 2008); suggesting an impairment in oxygen extraction at the muscle tissue level. Matsumoto *et al.* (2006) observed indications for an impaired mitochondrial oxygen consumption and a reduced oxygen delivery to the muscle in patients with ESRD using Near Infrared Spectroscopy (NIRS).

The objective of this study was to evaluate the cardiopulmonary exercise test (CPET) results in children with ESRD and compare their results with those of children with an acquired myopathy.

22.2 METHODS

Patients (13 boys and 7 girls; mean age 14.1±3.4 years) on dialysis (11 haemodialysis and 9 peritoneal dialysis) from four paediatric dialysis centres participated in this study. Their characteristics are described previously (Takken *et al.*, 2009). CPET was performed using a graded exercise test on a cycle ergometer (Lode Corrival pediatric) and a calibrated respiratory gas-analysis system (Cortex

MetaMax) to determine oxygen uptake ($\dot{V}O_{2peak}$), carbondioxide production ($\dot{V}CO_{2peak}$), Respiratory Exchange Ratio (RER_{peak}), ventilation ($\dot{V}_{Epeak}$), work rate (W_{peak}), and peak heart rate (HR_{peak}). Normative values were obtained from healthy Dutch peers (Binkhorst et al., 1992).

22.3   RESULTS

All patients were able to perform the exercise test without complications. One patient terminated the test prematurely because of breathing difficulties through the facemask. Therefore, we excluded this patient's exercise testing data from the analysis. The main reason for ending the exercise test was muscle fatigue in 19 patients.

Mean results are presented in Table 22.1. Mean HR_{peak} (168.67±22.78 (range 131-201 beats/min) was significantly lower compared with healthy reference values (P<0.001). The RER_{peak} was 1.15±0.15 (range 0.87-1.44). Eighty-five percent of the patients showed a reduction in $\dot{V}O_{2peak}/kg$ of >2 standard deviations below normal. Data concerning $\dot{V}O_2$, $\dot{V}O_{2peak}/kg$, $\dot{V}_{Epeak}$ and W_{peak} were significantly reduced compared with healthy reference values. Furthermore, the mean ventilatory threshold (VT) was 32.66% of predicted $\dot{V}O_{2peak}$, which is reduced as well. Ventilatory equivalent for oxygen ($\dot{V}_{Epeak}/\dot{V}O_{2peak}$) tended to be higher in children with ESRD compared with healthy reference values (37.9±7.0 and 35.7±2.4; p=0.18). Ventilatory equivalent for carbon dioxide ($\dot{V}_{Epeak}/\dot{V}CO_{2peak}$) was significantly higher in ESRD compared with healthy reference values (32.6±4.4 and 29.7±2.4; p=0.012). The average peak oxygen pulse ($\dot{V}O_{2peak}/HR_{peak}$) was 8.03±2.96 ml/beat which was 67.14±17.39% of predicted. No significant associations were found between exercise-related measurements and the time on dialysis or disease duration. All CPET characteristics were comparable with children with inflammatory myositis (Takken et al., 2008), except for $\dot{V}O_{2peak}/kg$ and W_{peak}, which where somewhat higher.

Table 22.1. Cardiopulmonary exercise test characteristics of children with ESRD compared with inflammatory myositis.

Parameter	ESRD Mean±SD	ESRD Predicted %	Myositis Mean±SD	Myositis Predicted %	p
$\dot{V}O_{2peak}$ (l/min)	1.34 ± 0.56	57.3 ± 14.5	1.0 ± 0.21	47.8 ± 13.9	0.07
$\dot{V}O_{2peak}/kg$ (ml/kg/min)	30.9 ± 6.99	66 ± 12	26.4 ± 8.9	55.1 ± 17.1	0.04
$\dot{V}O_{2peak}/HR_{peak}$	8.03 ± 2.96	67.1 ± 17.4	5.7 ± 1.4	61 ± 17.9	0.34
W_{peak} (Watt)	111.0 ± 48.3	54.4 ± 17	63 ± 23.8	40.9 ± 15.7	0.03
HR_{peak} (Beats/min)	168.4 ± 22.8	86.3 ± 12.1	175 ± 19.7	89 ± 10.1	0.67
VT as % of pred $\dot{V}O_{2peak}$	32.66 ± 8.86	55 ± 15	36.2 ± 13.1	56 ± 20	0.87

22.4 DISCUSSION

Children with ESRD have cardiopulmonary exercise test characteristics indicating a severely reduced exercise capacity. Their characteristics where in general comparable with those from children with inflammatory myositis (Takken *et al.*, 2008). A severe impairment of the exercise capacity was found in children with ESRD compared with healthy controls. This is in line with previous studies in children (Eijsermans *et al.*, 2004; Matsumoto *et al.*, 2006; Pattaragarn *et al.*, 2004) and adults with ESRD (Painter *et al.*, 2007). No relationship was found between time on dialysis or disease duration and exercise capacity. This suggests that even a short period of loss of renal function results in a severe reduced exercise capacity. Probable causes for this impairment might be inflammation, uremia, anaemia and cachexia. Moreover, inactivity may also attribute to the reduced exercise capacity (Krasnoff *et al.*, 2006).

There are two important determinants of $\dot{V}O_{2peak}$, central factors that control the delivery of oxygen to the skeletal muscle and the capacity of the skeletal muscle to extract and use oxygen for ATP production during exercise. In healthy subjects, the delivery of oxygen limits $\dot{V}O_{2peak}$ which means that the capacity to extract and use oxygen is greater than the capacity to deliver oxygen. In our patient group we found implications in the opposite direction. The characteristics of the CPET were similar to those observed in children with myositis. Therefore, it is reasonable to assume that the capacity of the skeletal muscle to extract and use oxygen is affected in ESRD. Previous studies in children with ESRD are supporting this finding (Matsumoto *et al.*, 2006, Miro *et al.*, 2002). Moreover, the peak heart rate during exercise was significantly lower in the present study compared with healthy children, although only 4 patients used antihypertensive drugs that blunted the heart rate response. Thus, the lower HR_{peak} in this patient group might be explained by the increased levels of leg muscle fatigue during exercise and this forced them to stop before cardio-pulmonary limitation. Thus, peripheral factors might limit the exercise capacity before central factors (cardiac output) reaches its limits. This is emphasized by low RER_{peak} values in some of our patients. It should be mentioned that RER_{peak} values might also be influenced by metabolic acidosis which is often present in ESRD. The increased peak ventilatory equivalent for carbon dioxide is an indicator of a gas-exchange abnormality. This might be caused by some anatomical thorax abnormalities in some patients. A reduced thoracic volume can be caused by growth restrictions and by the peritoneal fluid in case of peritoneal dialysis. Normally, activities of daily living are about 50% of $\dot{V}O_{2peak}$ which is no problem to perform over a sustained period of time. Children with a very low $\dot{V}O_{2peak}$ and VT could have problems with these activities, because their VT is lower than the oxygen cost of most activities of daily living.

Interventions targeting the exercise capacity seems indicated for pediatric ESRD patients. However, we and others have found that the feasibility of exercise training programs are limited in this patient group (Goldstein and Montgomery, 2009; van Bergen *et al.*, 2009). Drug treatment for additional capilarization in the muscle or improved mitochondrial function might be worthwhile to explore.

22.5   ACKNOWLEDGEMENTS

This study was funded by a grant from the Dutch Kidney Foundation (grant #KI30).

22.6   REFERENCES

Bar-Or, O. and Rowland, T.W., 2004, Pediatric Exercise Medicine. From physiologic principles to healthcare application. Champaign, IL: Human Kinetics.

Binkhorst, R.A., van't Hof, M.A. and Saris, W.H.M., 1992, Maximale inspanning door kinderen; referentiewaarden voor 6-18 jarige meisjes en jongens [Maximal exercise in children; reference values girls and boys, 6-18 year of age]. Den-Haag: Nederlandse Hartstichting.

Eijsermans, R.M., Creemers, D.G., Helders, P.J. and Schroder, C.H., 2004, Motor performance, exercise tolerance, and health-related quality of life in children on dialysis. *Pediatric Nephrology*, **19**, pp. 1262–1266.

Goldstein, S.L. and Montgomery, L.R., 2009, A pilot study of twice-weekly exercise during hemodialysis in children. *Pediatric Nephrology*, **24**, pp. 833–839.

Krasnoff, J.B., Mathias, R., Rosenthal, P. and Painter, P.L., 2006, The comprehensive assessment of physical fitness in children following kidney and liver transplantation. *Transplantation*, **82**, pp. 211–217.

Matsumoto, N., Ichimura, S., Hamaoka, T., Osada, T., Hattori, M. and Miyakawa, S., 2006, Impaired Muscle Oxygen Metabolism in Uremic Children: Improved After Renal Transplantation. *American Journal of Kidney Diseases*, **48**, pp. 473–480.

Miro, O., Marrades, R.M., Roca, J., Sala, E., Masanes, F., Campistol, J.M., Torregrosa, J.V., Casademont, J., Wagner, P.D. and Cardellach, F., 2002, Skeletal muscle mitochondrial function is preserved in young patients with chronic renal failure. *American Journal of Kidney Diseases*, **39**, p. 1025–1031.

Painter, P., Krasnoff, J. and Mathias, R., 2007, Exercise capacity and physical fitness in pediatric dialysis and kidney transplant patients. *Pediatric Nephrolology*, 22, pp. 1030–1039.

Painter, P., 2008, Exercise in chronic disease: physiological research needed. *Exercise and Sport Science Reviews*, **36**, pp. 83–90.

Pattaragarn, A., Warady, B.A. and Sabath, R.J, 2004, Exercise capacity in pediatric patients with end-stage renal disease. *Peritoneal Dialysis International*, **24**, pp. 274–80.

Robertson, H.T., Haley, N.R., Guthrie, M., Cardenas, D., Eschbach, J.W. and Adamson, J.W., 1990, Recombinant erythropoietin improves exercise capacity in anemic hemodialysis patients. *American Journal of Kidney Diseases*, **15**, pp. 325–332.

Takken, T., van der Net, J., Engelbert, R.H., Pater, S. and Helders, P.J., 2008, Responsiveness of exercise parameters in children with inflammatory myositis. *Arthritis and Rheumatism*, **59**, pp. 59–64.

Takken, T., Engelbert, R., van Bergen, M., Groothoff, J., Nauta, J., van Hoeck, K., Lilien, M. and Helders, P., 2009, Six-minute walking test in children with ESRD: discrimination validity and construct validity. *Pediatric Nephrology*, **24**, pp. 2217–2223.

Van Bergen, M., Takken, T., Engelbert, R., Groothoff, J., Nauta, J., van Hoeck, K., Helders, P. and Lilien, M., 2009, Exercise training in pediatric patients with end-stage renal disease. *Pediatric Nephrology*, **24**, pp. 619–622.

Warady, B.A., Sabath, R.J., Smith, C.A., Alon, U. and Hellerstein, S., 1991, Recombinant human erythropoietin therapy in pediatric patients receiving long-term peritoneal dialysis. *Pediatric Nephrology*, **5**, 718–723.

Muscle Oxidative Metabolism in Children and Adults during Moderate Intensity Cycling Exercise

E. Leclair[1], S. Berthoin[1], B. Borel[1], H. Carter[2], F. Prieur[3], D. Thevenet[4], G. Baquet[1], and P. Mucci[1]

[1]University of Lille 2, EA 4488, France; [2]University of Brighton, UK; [3]University of Lievin, France; [4]University of Rennes 2, France

23.1 INTRODUCTION

During moderate intensity exercise (intensity below ventilatory threshold), pulmonary oxygen uptake ($\dot{V}O_2$) is classically described by two phases. $\dot{V}O_2$ phase 2 is known to closely represent muscular O_2 consumption (Barstow and Molo, 1987). In spite of contradictory literature, some studies demonstrated that younger children displayed a faster $\dot{V}O_2$ phase 2 than adults (Armon *et al.*, 1991). This faster adjustment may be explained by a greater O_2 extraction at the muscle level during exercise. However this statement has never been assessed.

The Near Infrared Spectroscopy (NIRS) has the advantage to assess muscle oxygenation indexes which are the result of the balance (or unbalance) between O_2 delivery and O_2 extraction in the portion of tissue under consideration. More specifically, deoxygenation kinetics assessed with NIRS during exercise reflect muscle O_2 extraction (DeLorey *et al.*, 2004).

The aim of the study was to examine the temporal relationship between muscle O_2 consumption, as reflected by the $\dot{V}O_2$ phase 2, and deoxygenation of the vastus lateralis muscle measured with NIRS during moderate intensity constant load cycling exercise in children and adults

23.2 METHODS

23.2.1 Experimental design

Eleven prepubertal boys and 12 men, untrained and non-obese, volunteered to participate in the study. They performed on cycle-ergometer a maximal graded exercise to determine the power associated to ventilatory threshold (PVT) and four constant load exercises at 90% of PVT. During each trial, $\dot{V}O_2$ (Ergocard,

Medisoft) and muscle deoxygenation characterized by HHb signal (Oxymon, Artinis Medical system BV) were continuously monitored. $\dot{V}O_2$ phase 2 and HHb kinetics were modelled and characterized by time to achieve 63% of the phase amplitude (τ) and 63% of the overall signal (mean response time – MRT) respectively.

23.2.2 Pulmonary oxygen uptake

During all the tests, adults and children breathed through an adult or pediatric mask of low dead space adapted to their face. Respiratory gas-exchanges were measured breath-by-breath using an automated gas analysis system to determine ventilation, oxygen uptake ($\dot{V}O_2$), and carbon dioxide output.

23.2.3 Near infrared spectroscopy

During exercise, the NIRS probe was firmly attached to the skin overlying the lower third of the *vastus lateralis* muscle, parallel to the major axis of the thigh. A 4cm distance was kept between the optodes which were housed in a plastic holder, thus ensuring that the position of the optodes, relative to each other, was fixed and invariant.

NIRS is based on the relative tissue transparency for light in the near-infrared region and on the oxygen-dependent absorption changes of hemoglobin and myoglobin. By using a continuous wave near-infrared spectrophotometer that generates light at 905, 850 and 770 nm, it is possible to differenciate between oxy- and deoxy-hemoglobin/myoglobin (O_2Hb/O_2Mb and HHb/HMb, respectively).

Data were sampled at 10Hz from the beginning to the end of the exercise session, displayed real-time and stored for offline analysis.

23.2.4 Modelling procedures

$\dot{V}O_2$ and HHb data were interpolated to give second-by-second values. The four transitions were time aligned to the start of exercise and averaged to yield a single response for each subject. Nonlinear regression techniques were used to fit data with a monoexponential model and an iterative process ensured the sum of squared error was minimized.

The $\dot{V}O_2$ phase 2 was modelled after a time delay (TD) of 15s (Springer *et al.*, 1991), as follows:

$\dot{V}O_2$ (t) = $\dot{V}O_2$ (b) + Ax(1 – e [- (t-TD/τ)])   (DeLorey *et al.*, 2004)

The HHb data (ie. muscular deoxygenation) were modelled as follows:
   HHb(t) = HHb(b) + Ax(1 – e [- (t-TD/τ)])   (DeLorey *et al.*, 2004)
Where HHb(t) represents HHb at any time (t), HHb(b) is the baseline value of HHb before the onset of exercise, A is the amplitude of the increase in HHb above the baseline value, TD is the time delay before HHb increase above preexercise values,

and τ is the time constant defined as the duration of time through which HHb increases to a value equivalent to 63% of A.

Experimental data are presented as means ± standard deviations (mean ±SD). Mean values comparisons between children and adults were made with the Student's t test after verification for distribution normality. In all analysis, the level of significance was set at p<0.05.

23.3 RESULTS

Anthropometric characteristics and maximal graded test parameters are presented on Table 23.1. No significant difference in $\dot{V}O_2$max related to body mass between children and adults. The $\dot{V}O_2$ kinetics and NIRS derived parameters at the onset of exercise are presented on Table 23.2. For $\dot{V}O_2$ as for HHb, the kinetics responses were significantly faster in children when compared with adults.

Table 23.1. Anthropometric characteristics and maximal graded test parameters.

	n	Age (Years)	Height (cm)	Body mass (kg)	$\dot{V}O_2$max (ml.kg^{-1}.min^{-1})	PVT (W.kg^{-1})
Children	11	10.3±0.9	142.3±7.7	38.6±10.2	42.8±4.7	2.0+0.3
Adults	12	23.9±3.9	177.0±6.5	71.5±10.0	46.6±5.9	2.5±0.3

Table 23.2. Mean values of modelling parameters for $\dot{V}O_2$p and HHb in children and adults at onset of moderate intensity cycling exercise

	$\dot{V}O_2$p			HHb		
	TD (s)	τ (s)	MRT (s)	TD (s)	τ (s)	MRT (s)
Children	11	11.6±3.5	26.6±3.5	8.7±1.1	49.0±19.0	13.5±1.4
Adults	12	24.9±4.2***	39.9±4.2***	10.3±3.7	10.2±6.2**	20.3±6.8***

$\dot{V}O_2$: pulmonary oxygen uptake; HHb: deoxyhemoglobin; TF: time delay; τ: time constant; MRT: mean response time.
**: Significantly different from children at p<0.01
***: Significantly different from children at p<0.001

23.4 CONCLUSION

Our results confirmed previous results by Fawkner *et al.* (2002) showing a significantly (p<0.001) faster $\dot{V}O_2$ phase 2 in children compared to adults. In addition, we observed that following a similar time delay in children and adults, HHb adjustment (τ) at the exercise onset was almost two fold faster in children than in adults. The markedly faster muscle deoxygenation in children suggests that there was a greater mismatch between muscle O_2 delivery and muscle O_2 extraction during the moderate intensity exercise thereby indicating a greater O_2 extraction. In agreement with previous results, HHb mean response time (MRT =

TD + τ) was significantly shorter in children, indicating that the whole HHb response was faster in children.

These results (faster $\dot{V}O_2$ adjustment) support the hypothesis of an enhanced oxidative metabolism in children as compared with adults, which could be explained in part by an enhanced O_2 muscular extraction (faster HHb adjustment) during exercise.

23.5   REFERENCES

Armon, Y., Cooper, D.M., Flores, R., Zanconato, S. and Barstow, T.J., 1991, Oxygen uptake dynamics during high-intensity exercise in children and adults. *Journal of Applied Physiology*, **70**, pp. 841-848.

Barstow, T.J. and Mole, P.A., 1987, Simulation of pulmonary O_2 uptake during exercise transients in humans. *Journal of Applied Physiology*, **63**, pp. 2253-2261.

DeLorey, D.S., Kowalchuk, J.M. and Paterson, D.H., 2004, Effect of age on O_2 uptake kinetics and the adaptation of muscle deoxygenation at the onset of moderate-intensity cycling exercise. *Journal of Applied Physiology*, **97**, pp. 165-172.

DeLorey, D.S., Kowalchuk, J.M. and Paterson, D.H., 2004, Effects of prior heavy-intensity exercise on pulmonary O_2 uptake and muscle deoxygenation kinetics in young and older adult humans. *Journal of Applied Physiology*, **97**, pp. 998-1005.

Fawkner, S.G., Armstrong, N., Potter, C.R. and Welsman, J.R., 2002, Oxygen uptake kinetics in children and adults after the onset of moderate-intensity exercise. *Journal of Sports Sciences*, **204**, pp. 319-326.

Springer, C., Barstow, T.J., Wasserman, K. and Cooper, D.M., 1991, Oxygen uptake and heart rate responses during hypoxic exercise in children and adults. *Medicine and Science in Sports Exercise*, **23**, pp. 71-79.

CHAPTER NUMBER 24

Effect of Pedal Rate on Pulmonary Oxygen Uptake Kinetics during High-Intensity Cycling in Adolescent Boys

B.C. Breese, A.R. Barker, N. Armstrong, and C.A. Williams

Children's Health and Exercise Research Centre, School of Sport and Health
Sciences, University of Exeter, UK

24.1 INTRODUCTION

During high-intensity exercise (above the lactate threshold, T_{lac}) the O_2 cost of exercise is less 'efficient' due, in part, to a delayed-onset $\dot{V}O_2$ slow component (SC) that elevates oxygen uptake ($\dot{V}O_2$) above the predicted value extrapolated from the sub-T_{lac} $\dot{V}O_2$ - work rate relationship (Jones and Poole, 2005; Whipp and Wasserman, 1972). Since this 'excess' $\dot{V}O_2$ is reported to result in greater utilisation of finite phosphocreatine (PCr) (Rossiter et al., 2002) and glycogen reserves (Krustrup et al., 2004a), understanding the origin of the SC is of practical importance in terms of studying developmental aspects of muscle metabolism and exercise tolerance.

A recent study reported depletion of muscle PCr and glycogen from type II fibre pools exclusively at exercise work rates that elicited a $\dot{V}O_2$ SC (Krustrup et al., 2004b). Moreover, it might be expected that the recruitment of type II fibres would be further enhanced for the same external power output by increasing pedal rate based on skeletal muscle power-velocity relationships (Sargeant, 1994).

Therefore, the aim of this study was to investigate the mechanistic basis for the $\dot{V}O_2$ SC in adolescent boys using disparate pedal rates to alter muscle fibre recruitment patterns during high-intensity exercise. Given the potential for training status to modulate $\dot{V}O_2$ response dynamics (Koppo et al., 2004), we also sought to examine the influence of aerobic fitness on $\dot{V}O_2$ kinetics at high and low pedal rates in this age group.

24.2   METHODS

24.2.1 Participants

Seven junior cyclists (mean age: 16.3 ± 0.9 yr) and seven physically active teenage boys (mean age: 15.2 ± 0.8 yr) volunteered to participate in this study. The cyclists had all competed in national junior competition over the preceding 12 months. Written, informed consent was obtained from each participant and their parents prior to the commencement of the study after verbal and written explanations of the study's aims, risks, and procedures were provided.

24.2.2 Experimental procedures

During all exercise tests, gas-exchange variables were measured and displayed online by use of an EX670 mass spectrometer and analysis suite (Morgan Medical, Rainham, UK). On each of the first two visits subjects completed a ramp incremental test to voluntary exhaustion at a pedal rate of either 50 rpm or 115 rpm for determination of the cadence-specific peak $\dot{V}O_2$ and the gas exchange threshold (GET). The work rates that would require 70% of the difference (Δ) between the cadence-specific GET and peak $\dot{V}O_2$ were estimated for each cadence. On each of the subsequent two visits subjects performed two bouts of high-intensity exercise (70% Δ) at alternate pedal rates interspersed with 60-min recovery.

24.2.3 Data analysis

The breath-by-breath $\dot{V}O_2$ data from each 'step' exercise linearly interpolated to provide second-by-second values and, for each individual, identical repetitions of each rest-to-exercise transition were time aligned to the start of exercise and averaged together to form a single data set for analysis. After removal of phase I of the response, a single-exponential equation of the form described in Equation (1.1) was used to model the phase II response within a pre-determined fitting window that excluded the slow component.

$$\Delta \dot{V}O_2(t) = A \cdot (1 - e^{-(t-\delta)/\tau}) \text{ (phase } 1 < t < 360 \text{ s)} \qquad (1.1)$$

The amplitude of the slow component (A_s') was calculated as the difference in the mean of the $\dot{V}O_2$ amplitude over the last 30 s of exercise ($\dot{V}O_2tot$) and A. The slow component was expressed in relative terms as the percentage contribution of A_s' to $\dot{V}O_2tot$. The functional 'gain' of the phase II $\dot{V}O_2$ response was computed by dividing the amplitude of the phase II response (A) by the change in work rate (ΔWR). This method was replicated to compute the functional gain of the entire response.

24.2.4 Statistical analysis

Repeated-measures ANOVA were performed to identify significant changes in response measures between both pedal rates (independent variable) and any training interaction (between-subjects variable). Statistical significance was set at the $p<0.05$ level.

24.3   RESULTS

Peak $\dot{V}O_2$ (L·min^{-1}) was significantly greater in cyclists compared to control subjects across both pedal rate conditions ($p<0.05$). There was a significant interaction between training status and pedal rate on the $\dot{V}O_2$ kinetics at exercise onset ($p<0.05$). No significant differences were found for the $\dot{V}O_2$ low component between both groups. Results are shown in Table 24.1 and Figure 24.1.

Table 24.1. Oxygen uptake responses during high-intensity exercise at disparate pedal rates in cyclists (CYC) and control (CON) subjects. Values are mean ± SD.

	CON		CYC	
	50 rpm	115 rpm	50 rpm	115 rpm
Peak VO$_2$ (L·min^{-1})	3.6 ± 0.7*	3.7 ± 1.0	4.4 ± 0.5	4.6 ± 0.7
Phase II time constant (s)	29 ± 6†	41 ± 13	30 ± 6	29 ± 8
Primary gain (mL^{-1}·min^{-1}·W)	11.6 ± 1.0$^#$	8.8 ± 1.2	10.9 ± 0.7$^#$	9.1 + 0.9
Relative slow component (%)	9 ± 3	11 + 6	13 + 3	15 ± 3
Overall gain (mL^{-1}·min^{-1}·W)	12.7 + 1.0$^#$	9.9 ± 1.2	12.6 ± 0.9$^#$	11.0 ± 1.2

*Significant between-group differences, $p<0.05$. $^#$Significant within-group pedal rate differences, $p<0.01$. †Significant interaction between pedal rate and training status, $p<0.05$.

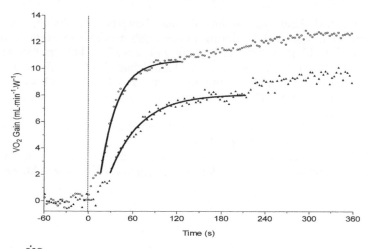

Figure 24.1. $\dot{V}O_2$ response during high-intensity exercise in a typical cyclist (○) and control subject (▲) pedalling at ~115 rpm. Solid black lines denote the model fit to the phase II response.

24.4   CONCLUSION

This study reported a significant slowing (~ 41%) of the $\dot{V}O_2$ kinetics at exercise-onset in adolescent boys during high-intensity cycling at an elevated pedal rate. These data presumably reflect the recruitment of type II muscle fibres with inherently slower $\dot{V}O_2$ kinetics as evidenced previously in animal muscle (Crow and Kushmerick, 1982). Since the rapidity in which muscle $\dot{V}O_2$ rises at exercise onset is intimately related to the O_2 deficit, the recruitment of these fibres has important implications on the utilisation of finite intramuscular energy stores and thus exercise tolerance in this population. No effect of pedal rate on phase II $\dot{V}O_2$ kinetics was found in junior cyclists of a similar age possibly due to specific training effects that enhance the mitochondrial O_2 utilisation potential in these same fibres.

24.5   REFERENCES

Crow, M. T. and Kushmerick, M.J., 1982, Chemical energetics of slow- and fast-twitch muscles of the mouse. *The Journal of General Physiology,* **79**, pp. 147–166.

Jones, A.M. and Poole, D.C., 2005, Oxygen uptake dynamics: from muscle to mouth—an introduction to the symposium. *Medicine and Science in Sports and Exercise,* **37**, pp. 1542–1550.

Koppo, K., Bouckaert, J. and Jones, A.M., 2004, Effects of training status and exercise intensity on phase II $\dot{V}O_2$ kinetics. *Medicine and Science in Sports and Exericise,* **36**, pp. 225–232.

Krustrup, P., Hellsten, Y. and Bangsbo, J., 2004a, Intense interval training enhances human skeletal muscle oxygen uptake in the initial phase of dynamic exercise at high but not at low intensities. *Journal of Physiology,* **559**, pp. 335–345.

Krustrup, P., Soderlund, K., Mohr, M. and Bangsbo, J., 2004b, The slow component of oxygen uptake during intense, sub-maximal exercise in man is associated with additional fibre recruitment. *Pflugers Arch,* **447**, pp. 855–866.

Rossiter, H. B., Ward, S. A., Howe, F. A., Kowalchuk, J. M., Griffiths, J. R. and Whipp, B. J., 2002, Dynamics of intramuscular ^{31}P-MRS P(i) peak splitting and the slow components of PCr and O_2 uptake during exercise. *Journal of Applied Physiology,* **93**, pp. 2059–2069.

Sargeant, A.J., 1994, Human power output and muscle fatigue. *International Journal of Sports Medicine,* **15**, pp. 116–121.

Whipp, B.J. and Wasserman, K., 1972, Oxygen uptake kinetics for various intensities of constant-load work. *Journal of Applied Physiology,* **33**, pp. 351–356.

Effects of Exercise Modality on Ventilatory Parameters in Prepubescent Children with Cystic Fibrosis

B. Borel[1], E. Leclair[1], D. Thevenet[2], L. Beghin[3-4], F. Gottrand[4], D. Turck[4], and C. Fabre[1]

[1]EA 4488, University of Lille 2, France; [2]M2S, ENS Cachan, University of Rennes 2, France; [3]CIC-9301-INSERM, CHRU of Lille, France; [4]U995, CHRU of Lille, France

25.1 INTRODUCTION

During training programs, the choice of the exercise modality is important for maintaining children's motivation at a high level and adhesion to physical activity. Even if continuous exercise modality is often used during training programs for children (McManus et al., 1997), it has been shown that this exercise modality could induce monotony and so could decrease the adhesion to physical activity in children with cystic fibrosis (Gulmans et al., 1999). Based on children's spontaneous physical activity pattern (Bailey et al., 1995), some studies have proposed training programs based on intermittent exercise modality (Baquet et al., 2002). However, compared to continuous modality, the intermittent modality could induce higher levels of ventilation as intermittent exercise is based on high exercise intensities. So, intermittent modality, even if it could be more pleasant for children, could be more difficult to bear in children with cystic fibrosis. To our knowledge, no study has focused on the effect of exercise modality on ventilatory response in prepubescent children with cystic fibrosis. As the ventilatory function is one of the most affected functions in cystic fibrosis, this type of information could be very useful in order to determine the most appropriate exercise modality for cystic fibrosis. Thus, the aim of the study was to compare ventilatory responses and mechanical ventilatory constraints following two exercise modalities (i.e. continuous vs. intermittent), at three intensity levels, in order to determine the benefits – risks of exercise on ventilatory function for children with cystic fibrosis (CF).

25.2   METHODS

25.2.1 Study design

Five prepubescent children with cystic fibrosis (age: 10.6 ± 1.5 years, forced expiratory volume in 1 second: 97.5 ± 16.8% of theoretical value) performed 7 tests on a treadmill during three different visits: an incremental test, 3 continuous and 3 intermittent exercises.

25.2.2 Exercise design

Invariably, children firstly performed a maximal graded test, with a 0.5km.h^{-1} increment per minute, in order to determine the maximal aerobic speed (MAS) of each child. MAS was used for individualizing the exercise intensities of the 6 other exercises. Continuous and intermittent exercises (CE and IE, respectively) were performed randomly and with 6-minute duration. IE consisted in the repetition of 15s of running periods intercepted by 15s of passive recovery periods. Intensities were fixed at 60%, 70% and 80% of measured MAS (CE60, CE70 and CE80 respectively) and at 90%, 100% and 110% of measured MAS for IE (IE90, IE100 and IE110 respectively).

25.2.3 Ventilatory parameters

During all the exercises, ventilation ($\dot{V}_E$), breathing frequency (*f*) and tidal volume (Vt) were measured breath by breath with a mouthpiece. Mechanical ventilatory constraints were evaluated by measuring exercise flow/volume loops (F/V loops). F/V loops were recorded during the first 30 seconds of the last minute of each exercise. So, intermittent design was modified during the last minute of exercise, with 30s period of running instead of 15s running period. Then, F/V loops were reported within the maximal flow/volume loop (MFVL) obtained at rest before each exercise. Expiratory flow limitation (expFL) was defined as the part of Vt that meets MFVL and expressed as % of Vt. Breathing strategy was evaluated by analyzing end-expiratory lung volume (EELV estimated from inspiratory capacity relative to vital capacity) and end-inspiratory lung volume (EILV estimated from Vt relative to inspiratory capacity). Dyspnea was evaluated immediately after the end of exercise with a modified CR-10 Borg's scale.

25.2.4 Statistical analysis

Standard statistical methods were used for the calculation of means and standard deviations. Normality was checked for each parameter with a Kolmogorov-Smirnov test. A two-way analysis of variance (modality by intensity) was used to evaluate the effect of exercise modality and intensity on breathing pattern and mechanical ventilatory constraints parameters. Multiple comparisons were made with the Bonferroni post-hoc test. In order to compare the ventilatory response depending on the exercise modality: continuous *vs.* intermittent, associations of exercises were paired according to an intensity level. So, three levels of exercise were created: low (CE60 *vs.* IE90), medium (CE70 *vs.* IE100), high (CE80 *vs.* IE110).

25.3   RESULTS

Mean MAS was 9.9 ± 2.1 km.h^{-1}. For each exercise modality, expiratory flow limitations (expFL) were highlighted, ranging between $8 - 91\%$ of Vt. For continuous *vs.* intermittent exercise comparison, no significant difference was found for ventilatory constraints: mean expFL, Vt/IC and IC/VC (Figure 25.1). For breathing pattern parameters (Table 25.1), only one significant difference was found, with higher $\dot{V}_E$ during IE90 than during CE60 (p=0.02). No significant difference was found within the three associations for dyspnea scores (Table 25.2).

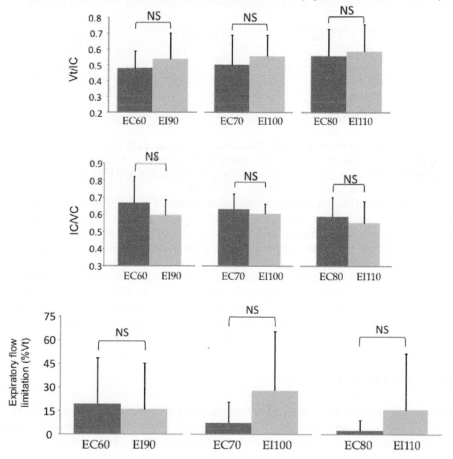

Figure 25.1. Mechanical ventilatory constraints during continuous and intermittent exercises depending on intensity levels. Values are mean ± SD.

Table 25.1. Breathing pattern during continuous and intermittent exercises depending on intensity levels. Values are mean ± SD.

	Low		Medium		High	
	CE60	IE90	CE70	IE100	CE80	IE110
Tidal Volume (L)	0.69±0.14	0.72±0.22	0.70±0.15	0.72±0.20	0.73±0.11	0.65±0.14
Breathing frequency (cycles.min^{-1})	45.3±6.5	56.3±9.3	55.7±16.3	60.7±11.0	63.9±13.4	69.9±13.3
Ventilation (L.min^{-1})	31.7±10.7	40.3±13.3*	38.4±13.3	43.2±10.3	46.5±12.8	45.8±15.4

* intra-association comparison: p=0.02

Table 25.2. Dyspnea scores at the end of continuous and intermittent exercises. Values are mean ± SD.

	Low		Medium		High	
	CE60	IE90	CE70	IE100	CE80	IE110
Dyspnea	0.40±0.42	0.50±0.35	0.80±0.82	1.30±1.57	2.30±1.64	1.70±1.99

25.4 CONCLUSION

The main finding of this study was that breathing patterns ($\dot{V}_E$, f, Vt) and mechanical ventilatory constraints parameters (expFL, EILV, EELV) were comparable whatever the exercise modality. However, during IE90, higher $\dot{V}_E$ was measured which could be due to higher f (p = 0.08).

Thus, intermittent and continuous exercises could be used for cystic fibrosis rehabilitation, allowing a diversification of physical activity programs and an enhancement of child adhesion to physical activity. The use of passive recovery could explain the prevention of the children from having a higher expiratory flow during intermittent exercise than during continuous exercise, making this mode of exercise acceptable for children, contrary to our first hypothesis. The acceptability of the intermittent exercise modality by the children is confirmed by dyspnea scores which are similar according to the intensity association. With passive recovery, intermittent exercises do not induce higher levels of ventilation. So, dyspnea scores are similar in both exercise modalities, as in COPD adult.

25.5 REFERENCES

Bailey, R.C., Olson, J., Pepper, S.L., Porszasz, J., Barstow, T.J. and Cooper, D.M., 1995, The level and tempo of children's physical activities: an observational study. *Medicine and Science in Sports and Exercise*, **27**, pp. 1033–1041.

Baquet, G., Berthoin, S., Dupont, G., Blondel, N., Fabre, C. and van Praagh, E., 2002, Effects of high intensity intermittent training on peak $\dot{V}O_2$ in prepubertal children. *International Journal of Sports Medicine*, **23**, pp. 439–444.

Gulmans, V.A., de Meer, K., Brackel, H.J., Faber, J.A., Berger, R. and Helders, P.J., 1999, Outpatient exercise training in children with cystic fibrosis: physiological effects, perceived competence, and acceptability, *Pediatric Pulmonology*, **28**, pp. 39–46.

McManus, A.M., Armstrong, N. and Williams, C.A., 1997, Effect of training on the aerobic power and anaerobic performance of prepubertal girls. *Acta Paediatrica*, **86**, pp. 456–459.

Part V

Children's Performances

Part V

Children's Performances

Effect of Maturation on the Relationship between Muscle Size and Force Production

A. Tonson[1], S. Ratel[2], Y. Lefur[1], P. Cozzone[1], and D. Bendahan[1]

[1]University of the Mediterranean Aix-Marseille II, France; [2]University of Blaise Pascal, Clermont Ferrand II, France

26.1 INTRODUCTION

Although it is commonly accepted that muscle size determines the maximal isometric strength that a human skeletal muscle can produce in healthy adults regardless of the sex, it is unclear whether this relationship changes during growth and maturation. Results reported in pediatric populations are highly controversial. The ratio of isometric strength to maximal muscle cross sectional area (MCSA) has been reported as unchanged throughout adolescence and early adulthood in elbow flexors and triceps surae muscle (Davies et al., 1983; Ikai and Fukunaga, 1968), whereas a significant increase has been reported during growth for isometric and dynamic exercises (Halin et al., 2003; Kenehisa et al., 1995; Saavedra et al., 1991). However, part of these controversies could be attributed to methodological discrepancies among the studies. More particularly, precise quantification of muscle volume or maximal muscle cross sectional area (MCSA) from anthropometric measurements might not be as accurate in children as it is in adults.

The main purpose of this study was to determine whether the relationship between muscle size and maximum isometric strength did change during growth and maturation. In addition to that, we quantified the potential measurements bias introduced by anthropometric estimations of local muscle volume considering MRI as the gold standard technique. We also determined the differences when muscle size was estimated from volume and MCSA measurements in a paediatric population.

26.2 METHODS

26.2.1 Subjects

45 healthy subjects were included in the present study, 14 pre-pubertal boys (11.3 ± 0.7 y.o., Tanner's stages ranging from 1 to 2) 16 pubertal boys (13.3 ± 1.4 y.o., Tanner's stages ranging from 3 to 4) and 15 men (35.4 ± 6.4 y.o.). The stages of pubertal development were determined from pubic hair and genital development (Tanner and Whitehouse, 1976).

26.2.2 Maximum voluntary isometric force measurement

The maximal isometric digitorum flexor strength (F_{max}) was measured using a dedicated experimental setup including a force transducer (ZF 100, Scaime, France) connected to a handle bar. F_{max} was defined as the mean of three reproducible measurements and the specific force corresponded to this value related to muscle size. Each measurement was performed after 1 min resting period. The variability of each trial was 3.0 ± 2.2 % whatever the age.

26.2.3 Anthropometric measurements

The forearm lean (muscle + bone) volume was determined from circumferences and skin-fold thickness measurements according to the Jones and Pearson method (Jones and Pearson, 1969).

26.2.4 MRI measurements

MRI investigations were performed at 1.5 T on a whole body Siemens –Vision Plus Imaging system (Siemens Germany).

The muscle volume (V_M) was quantified from T1-weighted images (9 to 13 slices depending on the forearm length) recorded with the following parameters (TR=490ms, TE=12ms, field of view=200mm, matrix: 512*512, slice thickness= 5mm and inter-slice gap=10mm). The cross sectional area of each slice was determined using an IDL (Interactive Data Language, RSI) home-written routine (Mattei *et al.*, 2006). Briefly, on the basis of a signal intensity threshold, fat, muscle and bone signals were clearly separated and quantified. Muscle volume (V_M) was calculated by summing all the slices area taking into account the slice thickness and the inter-slide space.

The anatomical maximal cross sectional area (MCSA) was defined as the highest area measured among different slices.

26.2.5 Statistical analysis

All results were expressed as means and standard deviations (mean ± SD). Each variable distribution has been tested and appropriate one-way ANOVA was used in order to compare the three groups. If the first test provided a significant difference, then each group was compared to the other two using post-hoc Tukey-Kramer tests. Relationships between variables were analysed using linear regressions and the corresponding strength was assessed using Pearson's correlation coefficient. The limit for statistical significance was set at $P<0.05$.

26.3 RESULTS

Forearm muscle volume determined from MRI (V_M) or anthropometric (V_L) measurements was significantly higher in adults than in children and adolescents (Table 26.1). Similarly, F_{max} significantly increased with respect to age from 174.9 ± 31.8 N in children to 456.2 ± 49.2 N in men.

Moreover, F_{max} was positively and linearly correlated to muscle size whatever the index chosen, i.e., MCSA ($F_{max} = 11.9$ MCSA $- 41.1$, $r^2 = 0.87$ and $P< 0.001$), muscle volume estimated by anthropometry ($F_{max} = 0.81$ $V_L - 77.0$, $r^2 = 0.85$, $P< 0.001$) or measured by MRI ($F_{max} = 0.83$ V_M, $r^2 = 0.90$ $P< 0.001$). Related to this latter index, the specific force was similar whatever the age (Table 26.2). On the contrary, the maximal force scaled to MCSA or muscle volume estimated by anthropometry, was significantly lower in children and adolescents than in men.

In addition, we observed a strong linear relationship between muscle volume measured by MRI and estimated by anthropometry ($V_L = 0.99$ $V_M + 107.3$, $r^2 = 0.90$ and $P< 0.001$). However, the forearm muscle volume calculated from anthropometric measurements (V_L) was systematically overestimated with respect to MRI muscle volume values (V_M). More importantly, the overestimation was significantly larger in children and adolescents as compared to adults (43.1 ± 15.2%; 38.5 ± 18.8% and 20.5± 10.5 % respectively).

Table 26.1. Specific force measurements.

	Children	Adolescents	Adults
$F_{max}.V_M^{-1}$, N.cm^{-3}	0.82 ± 0.2 *	0.80 ± 0.1 §	0.86 ± 0.1
$F_{max}.V_L^{-1}$, N.cm^{-3}	0.58± 0.1 *	0.58 ± 0.1 §	0.71 ± 0.1
$F_{max}.MCSA^{-1}$, N.cm^{-2}	9.45 ± 1.6 *	9.74 ± 2.0 §	11.3 ± 7.3

Values are presented as means ± standard deviation for all groups.
F_{max}: maximal isometric force of the flexors digitorum muscles; V_M, muscle forearm volume measured using MRI; V_L: forearm lean (muscle + bone) volume determined by anthropometry.
* and § refer to significant differences ($P< 0.05$) between children and adults and between adolescents and adults respectively.

Table 26.2. Specific force measurements.

	Children	Adolescents	Adults
$F_{max}.V_M^{-1}$, N.cm^{-3}	0.82 ± 0.2	0.80 ± 0.1	0.85 ± 0.1
$F_{max}.V_L^{-1}$, N.cm^{-3}	0.58 ± 0.1 *	0.58 ± 0.1 *	0.71 ± 0.1
$F_{max}.MCSA^{-1}$, N.cm^{-2}	9.45 ± 1.6 *	9.74 ± 2.0 *	11.3 ± 7.3

Values are presented as means ± standard deviation for all groups.

F_{max}: maximal isometric force of the flexors digitorum muscles; V_M, muscle forearm volume measured using MRI; V_L: forearm lean (muscle + bone) volume determined by anthropometry. * refers to significant differences ($P< 0.05$) with adults .

26.4   CONCLUSION

We have clearly demonstrated in the present study that the method used to quantify muscle size can influence the relationship between muscle size and force and more importantly the associated interpretation regarding changes during growth and maturation.

Using a reliable index of muscle size our results clearly showed that the force production ability is mainly determined by muscle size whatever the age.

The increase in the strength capacity previously reported during growth is likely due to inaccuracies related to muscle size measurements rather than biochemical or neural changes related to maturation.

26.5   REFERENCES

Davies, C.T., White, M.J. and Young, K., 1983, Muscle function in children. *European Journal of Applied Physiology and Occupational Physiology*, **52**, pp. 111–114.

Halin, R., Germain, P., Bercier, S., Kapitaniak B. and Buttelli O., 2003, Neuromuscular response of young boys versus men during sustained maximal contraction. *Medicine and Science in Sports and Exercise*, **35**, pp. 1042–1048.

Ikai, M. and Fukunaga, T., 1968, Calculation of muscle strength per unit cross-sectional area of human muscle by means of ultrasonic measurement. *International Zeitung Angewandte Physiologie*, **26**, pp. 26–32.

Jones, P.R. and Pearson, J., 1969, Anthropometric determination of leg fat and muscle plus bone volumes in young male and female adults. *Journal of Physiology*, **204**, pp. 63–66.

Kanehisa, H., Yata, H., Ikegawa, S. and Fukunaga, T.A., 1995, Cross-sectional study of the size and strength of the lower leg muscles during growth. *European Journal of Applied Physiology and Occupational Physiology*, **72**, pp. 150–156.

Mattei, J.P., Fur, Y.L., Cuge, N., Guis, S., Cozzone, P.J. and Bendahan, D., 2006, Segmentation of fascias, fat and muscle from magnetic resonance images in humans: the DISPIMAG software. *Magma*, **19**, pp. 275–279.

Saavedra, C., Lagasse, P., Bouchard, C. and Simoneau, J.A., 1991, Maximal anaerobic performance of the knee extensor muscles during growth. *Medicine and Science in Sports and Exercise*, **23**, pp. 1083–1089.

Tanner, J.M. and Whitehouse, R.H., 1976, Clinical longitudinal standards for height, weight, height velocity, weight velocity, and stages of puberty. *Archives of Disease in Childhood*, **51**, pp. 170–179.

Rate of Muscle Activation in Pre- and Early-Pubertal Power- and Endurance-Trained Male Athletes

B. Falk, R. Cohen, C. Mitchell, R. Dotan, P. Klentrou, and D. Gabriel

Faculty of Applied Health Sciences, Brock University, St Catharines, ON, Canada

27.1 INTRODUCTION

Power training has been demonstrated to result in enhanced muscle strength and explosive power in adults (Aagaard *et al.*, 2002). In children, power or high resistance training has been shown to result in enhanced maximal muscle strength (Behm *et al.*, 2008), but the possible effects on explosive strength are unknown. In adults, the enhanced muscle performance is a result of muscle hypertrophy, as well as neurological adaptations (Sale, 1988; Folland and Williams, 2007). In children, no muscle hypertrophy has been demonstrated as a result of resistance training (Behm *et al.*, 2008). Thus, it is assumed that muscle strength improvements are the result of neurological adaptations. Indeed, some evidence suggests greater motor unit recruitment in children as a result of resistance training (Ramsay *et al.*, 1990).

The effects of endurance training on muscle performance have been investigated to a limited extent in adults, demonstrating either no change (Hickson, 1980; Grandys *et al.*, 2008) or some enhancement in muscle maximal and explosive strength (Lattier *et al.*, 2003). Likewise, endurance training has been shown to be associated with some neural adaptations in adults (Lattier *et al.*, 2003). In children, the effects of endurance training on muscle performance, morphology or neural response has not been examined.

27.2 METHODS

27.2.1 Subjects

Eighteen untrained boys, 12 competitive swimmers, and 9 gymnasts volunteered to participate in the study. All subjects were at the pre- or early-pubertal stages (7-12 years old). Gymnasts had been training for 4.6±3.3 years. Swimmers had been

training for 2.5±0.9 years. The control subjects were involved in organized sports
for no more than 2 hr·wk-^{1}.

27.2.2 Procedure

Subjects made two visits to the laboratory, 2-7 days apart. During the first visit,
anthropometric measurements were taken (see measurements, below), and B-Mode
ultrasound was used to assess quadriceps and hamstrings muscle depth (diameter),
from which muscle cross sectional area (CSA) was calculated. The subjects were
then familiarized with the testing apparatus and procedures.

On their second visit, subjects performed a light specific warm-up and 10
maximal repetitions in each mode in a counterbalanced order. Following 2-3 min
rest, maximal repetitions were performed in two sets of 5 MVCs, 30 s apart, with a
2-min rest interval between sets. Subjects were asked to refrain from intense
physical activity for 48 hours prior to the experimental session.

27.2.3 Measurements

To estimate muscle diameter, muscle depth was measured using B-mode
ultrasound (System5, GE Vingmed, Horten, Norway), with 5 MHz linear-array
probe. The probe was placed over the bellies of the rectus femoris and biceps
femoris. Images were captured, stored and analyzed off-line. The muscle depth
was defined as the distance from the bone-muscle interface to the beginning of the
muscle-subcutaneous fat interface.

All strength testing was performed on a Biodex system 3 dynamometer. The
subjects were instructed to contract, from a relaxed state, "as fast and forcefully as
possible" so as to maximize torque and rate of torque development (RTD). They
were verbally encouraged throughout the testing session. In addition, all subjects
had online visual feedback of their torque signal on a PC screen. Isometric
contractions were chosen to minimize antagonist co-activation, so as to facilitate
attribution of torque measurements to agonist action.

Electrodes were placed parallel to the direction of the muscle fibres, on the
medial aspect of the vastus lateralis and on the belly of the biceps femoris. The
EMG signal was recorded using a Delsys (Boston, MA) Bagnoli EMG system and
bipolar DE-2.1 differential surface electrodes (1mm x 10mm Ag electrodes, 10mm
inter-electrode distance). The signal was then amplified 1000 times by a Bagnoli
amplifier (frequency response range 20-450 Hz, CMRR 92 dB). An analog-to-
digital (A-to-D) card was used to transfer the signal to a personal computer where
it was sampled at 1000 Hz, using Delsys EMGWorks acquisition software. The
torque signal from the Biodex was scaled to each subject's maximal torque and
transformed with the A-to-D.

Torque onset was defined as the first time point where the rate of torque
development (RTD) reached above 5 SD of the mean of the baseline for at least 10
ms. An average waveform was created by aligning the 5 best trials on their force
onset. The agonist and antagonist EMG signals were averaged to create average
waveforms, time-locked to the torque average waveform. The onset of EMG

activity was set at the point in time where the signal first increased 5 standard deviations above the mean of the baseline. The area under the rectified agonist EMG curve for the first 30 ms after the onset of EMG activity was defined as the Q_{30} (Gabriel and Boucher, 2000). Q_{30} was normalized to peak EMG amplitude to account for differences in signal amplitude due to factors such as muscle size, thickness of subcutaneous tissue or variations in electrode placement.

Electromechanical delay (EMD) was defined as the time lapse between the onsets of EMG and torque generation and calculated in the agonist muscle.

27.2.4 Statistical analysis

All data are displayed as mean ±1SD. All statistical analysis was conducted using SPSS 16.0.with α set at $p \leq 0.05$. Differences between means were compared using ANOVA. An LSD post hoc test was used to assess pair-wise differences.

27.3 RESULTS

When corrected for muscle CSA, no group differences were observed in peak extension strength (4.8 ± 1.9, 5.1 ± 1.1, and 3.8 ± 0.9 Nm.cm^{-2}, for controls, swimmers and gymnasts, respectively), or in peak flexion strength (2.2 ± 0.7, 2.5 ± 0.6, and 2.0 ± 0.5 Nm.cm^{-2}, respectively).

Figures 27.1 and 27.2 illustrate the mean peak RTD and Q_{30} for each group during knee extension and flexion. Gymnasts had significantly greater peak RTD, normalized to peak torque, during knee extension but not during knee flexion. The gymnasts' advantage was even greater for both raw and normalized Q_{30}.

EMD was significantly shorter EMD in power-athletes compared with controls (p=0.02) but not compared with endurance-trained athletes (p=0.24). No such differences were observed during knee flexion.

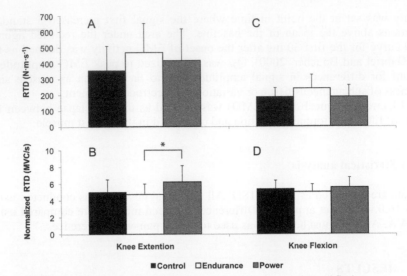

Figure 27.1. Mean peak RTD for each group during knee extension and flexion.

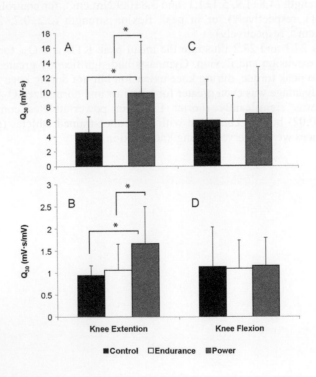

Figure 27.2. Mean peak Q_{30} for each group during knee extension and flexion.

27.4 CONCLUSION

This study examined maximal voluntary isometric torque and rate of torque development, along with the rate of muscle activation, during knee extension and flexion in muscle endurance-trained, power-trained and minimally active boys. The main findings were the greater rate of torque development, along with greater rate of muscle activation and lower EMD in the power-trained boys during knee extension but not during knee flexion. These findings suggest that, already during pre-adolescence, specific training can affect not only gross muscle performance capacity such as strength but the way muscles are activated, as well.

27.5 REFERENCES

Aagaard, P., Simonsen, E.B., Andersen, J.L., Magnusson, P. and Dyrhe-Poulsen, P., 2002, Increased rate of force development and neural drive of human skeletal muscle following resistance training. *Journal of Applied Physiology*, **93**, pp. 1318–1326.

Behm, D.G., Faigenbaum, A.D., Falk, B. and Klentrou, P., 2008, Canadian Society for Exercise Physiology position paper: resistance training in children and adolescents. *Applied Physiology Nutrition and Metabolism*, **33**, pp. 547–561.

Folland, J.P. and Williams, A.G. 2007, The adaptations to strength training: morphological and neurological contributions to increased strength. *Sports Medicine*, **37**, pp. 145–168.

Gabriel, D.A. and Boucher, J.P., 2000, Practicing a maximal performance task: a cooperative strategy for muscle activity. *Research Quarterly for Exercise and Sport*, **71**, pp. 217–228.

Grandys, M., Majerczak, J., Duda, K., Zapart-Bukowska, J., Sztzfko, K. and Zoladz, J.A., 2008, The effect of endurance training on muscle strength in young, healthy men in relation to hormonal status. *Journal of Physiology and Pharmacolology*, **59**, Suppl 7, pp. 89–103.

Hickson, R.C., 1980, Interference of strength development by simultaneously training for strength and endurance. *European Journal of Applied Physiology Occupational Physiology*, **45**, pp. 255–263.

Lattier, G., Millet, G.Y., Maffiuletti, N.A., Babault, N. and Candau, N., 2003, Neuromuscular differences between endurance-trained, power-trained, and sedentary subjects. *Journal of Strength and Conditioning Research*, **17**, pp. 514–521.

Ramsay, J.A., Blimkie, C.J., Smith, K., Garner S., MacDougall, J.D., and Sale, D.G., 1990, Strength training effects in prepubescent boys. *Medicine and Science in Sports and Exercise*, **22**, pp. 605–614.

Sale, D.G., 1988, Neural adaptation to resistance training. *Medicine and Science in Sports and Exercise*, **20**, pp. S135–145.

CHAPTER NUMBER 28

Recovery from Brief Isometric Calf Exercise in Young and Adult Females Measured with ^{31}P-MRS

R.J. Willcocks[1], J. Fulford[2], A.R. Barker[1], and C.A. Williams[1]

[1]School of Sport and Health Sciences, University of Exeter, Exeter, UK;
[2]Peninsula NIHR Clinical Research Facility, University of Exeter, Exeter, UK

28.1 INTRODUCTION

The speed of the monoexponential recovery of phosphocreatine (PCr) following exercise is determined by the oxidative capacity of the muscle (Meyer 1988; Paganini *et al.*, 1997). Oxidative capacity is an important measure of muscular fitness in healthy and unhealthy individuals, and is thought to be higher in children than adults (Taylor *et al.*, 1997; Ratel *et al.*, 2008), although contradictory evidence exists (Kuno *et al.*, 1995; Barker *et al.*, 2008). A measure of oxidative capacity in children could be used to investigate a number of questions related to the development of muscle function, including trainability, alterations in disease and with treatment, and maturational changes over time.

   Measurement of PCr recovery often requires participants to complete repeated exercise tests. The results of these tests are averaged to increase confidence in the parameters of the response (Barker *et al.*, 2008). The monoexponential recovery of PCr is then fitted with an exponential curve characterised by the time constant (τ). A set of recent studies have used a gated exercise protocol to measure the PCr recovery time constant in one test (Slade *et al.*, 2006; Forbes *et al.*, 2009). This type of protocol, which doesn't require sustained exercise or multiple tests, is well suited for use in a paediatric population. The purpose of this study was to evaluate a gated isometric exercise protocol to measure PCr recovery kinetics in 14 year old girls and adult women.

28.2 METHODS

Six girls (14 $\pm$ 0.2 y, 51.9 $\pm$ 9.0 kg, 1.61 $\pm$ 0.05 m, 1.4 $\pm$ 0.5 y past age at peak height velocity) and seven women (25 $\pm$ 3 years, 63.2 $\pm$ 5.5 kg, 1.65 $\pm$ 0.04 m) were recruited to participate in the study, which was approved by the institutional ethics committee. Calf muscle maximal voluntary contraction (MVC) was measured using a custom-built calf ergometer. Each participant completed a gated isometric exercise test within a 1.5 T magnetic resonance scanner. PCr and pH were measured every four seconds throughout exercise. Participants performed 23 contraction cycles (4 s maximal voluntary isometric calf contraction, 12 s recovery), and the final 18 contractions were included in analysis.

PCr values corresponding to the mean end-contraction PCr depletion (Q) and mean end-recovery PCr depletion (D) were calculated. These were analysed using equation 1 to give the PCr recovery time constant (see Figure 28.1).

$$\tau = -\Delta t/(\ln[D/(D+Q)])   \quad (1)$$

Intramuscular pH was averaged over the two minute resting baseline and each minute of exercise. Young and adult females were compared using independent t-tests, with significance accepted at $p \le 0.05$.

28.3   RESULTS

Calf muscle MVC in adolescent girls (431 ± 77 N) was significantly lower than in adult women (551 ± 43 N, p=0.01). Figure 28.1 shows the average PCr response to gated exercise in adolescent girls. The PCr recovery τ was similar in adolescent girls (20 ± 6 s) and women (20 ± 5 s, p=0.93). The steady state drop in PCr (D) was similar in adolescent girls (21 ± 4%) and women (18 ± 3%, p=0.27), as was the PCr cost of contraction (Q) (girls: 30 ± 11%, women: 24 ± 8%, p=0.39).

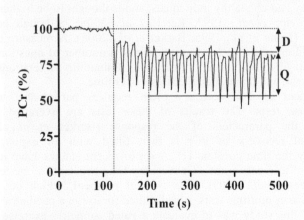

Figure 28.1. PCr during a graded exercise test in four girls. The onset of exercise and beginning of analysis are shown in dotted lines, and the parameters of the analysis are indicated (PCr is expressed as a percentage fall from baseline).

Intracellular pH estimates in this study should be interpreted with caution; poor signal-to-noise ratio in the spectra resulted in wide variation in the calculated pH at baseline and during exercise – the mean standard deviation in pH for each participant averaged across two minutes of rest was 0.23 in girls and 0.15 in women. However, qualitative inspection of the data revealed that pH increased at the onset of exercise in both groups, and thereafter appeared to decrease (though never below resting baseline) in girls while remaining constant in women.

28.4 DISCUSSION

The purpose of this study was to examine the feasibility of using a gated exercise protocol to determine oxidative capacity in a paediatric population. This technique was successfully used to determine a PCr recovery τ in four adolescent girls (67 % success) and seven women (100 % success). In two adolescent girls, poor signal-to-noise ratio prevented determination of the parameters of the response. There are several methods of increasing signal-to-noise ratio, including investigating a larger muscle group (such as the quadriceps), using a higher magnetic field strength scanner, or decreasing temporal resolution.

In this study, we examined PCr recovery kinetics in adolescent girls and women. Although investigation of maturational changes in PCr recovery was not an aim of the study, it was interesting to note that, in contrast with some previous investigations (Taylor *et al.*, 1997; Ratel *et al.*, 2008), but in keeping with others (Kuno *et al.*, 1995; Barker *et al.*, 2008), PCr recovery was not faster in young participants. This might be due to the advanced maturational status in the young girls, or might be due to close matching of exercise demand. PCr recovery is determined by mitochondrial function as well as the metabolic state at the end of exercise. Specifically, decreased intramuscular pH increases PCr recovery τ (Jubrias *et al.*, 2003; van den Broek *et al.*, 2007). End-exercise PCr might influence PCr recovery kinetics (Bendahan *et al.*, 2003), and resting [PCr] also affects the speed of PCr recovery (Meyer, 1988). While there might be differences in [PCr] in children and adults (Eriksson *et al.*, 1971), in this protocol, there was no decrease in intramuscular pH, and no difference between adolescent girls and women in the PCr cost of the exercise. The similar end-exercise muscle state in different groups is an important methodological feature of this protocol.

Gated exercise for the determination of oxidative capacity has many potential applications. A recent study has suggested that PCr recovery could be used as an indicator of insulin sensitivity in children (Fleischman *et al.*, 2009). A non-invasive, non-strenuous measure of oxidative capacity might also be desirable in studies examining training adaptations in children, maturational changes in mitochondrial function, and alterations in oxidative capacity with disease and treatment in children. Gated exercise offers a promising method of investigating muscle function in children.

28.5 REFERENCES

Barker, A.R., Welsman, J.R., Fulford, J., Welford, D. and Armstrong, N., 2008, Muscle phosphocreatine kinetics in children and adults at the onset and offset of moderate-intensity exercise. *Journal of Applied Physiology*, **105**, pp. 446–456.

Barker, A.R., Welsman, J.R., Fulford, J., Welford, D., Williams, C.A. and Armstrong, N., 2008, Muscle phosphocreatine and pulmonary oxygen uptake kinetics in children at the onset and offset of moderate intensity exercise. *European Journal of Applied Physiology and Occupational Physiology*, **102**, pp. 727–738.

Bendahan, D., Kemp, G.J., Roussel, M., Fur, Y.L. and Cozzone, P.J., 2003, ATP synthesis and proton handling in muscle during short periods of exercise and subsequent recovery. *Journal of Applied Physiology*, **94**, pp. 2391–2397.

Eriksson, B.O., Karlsson, J. and Saltin, B., 1971, Muscle metabolites during exercise in pubertal boys. *Acta Paediatrica Scandinavica.*, **217**, pp. S154–S157.

Fleischman, A., Kron, M., Systrom, D.M., Hrovat, M. and Grinspoon, S.K., 2009, Mitochondrial Function and Insulin Resistance in Overweight and Normal-Weight Children. *Journal of Clinical Endocrinology and Metabolism*, **99**, pp. 4923–4930.

Forbes, S.C., Slade, J.M., Francis, R.M. and Meyer, R.A., 2009, Comparison of oxidative capacity among leg muscles in humans using gated (31)P 2-D chemical shift imaging. *NMR in Biomedicine*, **22**, pp. 1063–1071.

Jubrias, S.A., Crowther, G.J., Shankland, E.G., Gronka, R.K. and Conley, K.E., 2003, Acidosis inhibits oxidative phosphorylation in contracting human skeletal muscle in vivo. *Journal of Physiology*, **553**, pp. 589–599.

Kuno, S., Takahashi, H., Fujimoto, K., Akima, H., Miyamaru, M., Nemoto, I., Itai, Y. and Katsuta, S., 1995, Muscle metabolism during exercise using phosphorus-31 nuclear magnetic resonance spectroscopy in adolescents. *European Journal of Applied Physiology and Occupational Physiology*, **70**, pp. 301–304.

Meyer, R.A., 1988, A linear model of muscle respiration explains monoexponential phosphocreatine changes. *American Journal of Physiology*, **254**, pp. C548–C553.

Paganini, A.T., Foley, J.M. and Meyer, R.A., 1997, Linear dependence of muscle phosphocreatine kinetics on oxidative capacity. *American Journal of Physiology*, **272**, pp. C501–C510.

Ratel, S., Tonson, A., Le Fur, Y., Cozzone, P. and Bendahan, D., 2008, Comparative analysis of skeletal muscle oxidative capacity in children and adults: a 31P-MRS study. *Applied Physiology Nutrition and Metabolism*, **33**, pp. 720–727.

Slade, J.M., Towse, T.F., Delano, M.C., Wiseman, R.W. and Meyer, R.A., 2006, A gated 31P NMR method for the estimation of phosphocreatine recovery time and contractile ATP cost in human muscle. *NMR in Biomedicine*, **19**, pp. 573–580.

Taylor, D.J., Kemp, G.J., Thompson, C.H. and Radda, G.K., 1997, Ageing: Effects on oxidative function of skeletal muscle in vivo. *Molecular and Cellular Biochemistry*, V174, pp. 321.

van den Broek, N.M.A., De Feyter, H.M.M.L., Graaf, L.d., Nicolay, K. and Prompers, J.J., 2007, Intersubject differences in the effect of acidosis on phosphocreatine recovery kinetics in muscle after exercise are due to differences in proton efflux rates. *American Journal of Physiology*, **293**, pp. C228–C237.

Anaerobic-to-Aerobic Power Ratio in Children with Juvenile Idiopathic Arthritis

M. Van Brussel[1], L. Van Doren[1], B.W. Timmons[2], J. Obeid[2], J. Van Der Net[1], P.J.M. Helders[1], and T. Takken[1]

[1]Wilhemina Children's Hospital, University Medical Center Utrecht, The Netherlands; [2]McMaster University and McMaster Children's Hospital, Hamilton, Ontario, Canada

29.1 INTRODUCTION

Children with Juvenile Idiopathic Arthritis (JIA) experience joint swelling, pain, and limited mobility, which contribute to decreased physical activity, fitness, and function (Klepper, 2003). This lower physical activity may lead to deconditioning and functional deterioration, which reinforces an inactive lifestyle (Takken et al., 2008). For example, most studies that measured the aerobic capacity of children with JIA (Takken et al., 2002; Metin et al., 2004, Van Brussel et al., 2007) have found reduced aerobic capacity. In addition, it has been found that these children present an impaired anaerobic capacity as well (Van Brussel et al., 2007). Limitations in anaerobic capacity might be caused by localized muscle weakness and atrophy around inflamed joints in children with JIA. Therefore, exercise therapy programs in the management of JIA are becoming increasingly important as these programs have been shown to prevent deconditioning and discontinue the vicious circle of inactivity and deteriorating functional ability reported in this population (Takken et al., 2008). Although the importance of exercise therapy in JIA is no longer disputed, prescribed exercise may vary considerably. A rationale for this variability is a lack of understanding as to whether exercise training should be more focused on aerobic or anaerobic exercise, or a combination of these energy systems. In addition, the evidence base for the prescription of exercise for children with JIA is rather small, and is based on 3 small randomized controlled trials (Takken et al., 2008). Given the described deficits in both aerobic and anaerobic exercise capacity in children with JIA (Van Brussel et al., 2007), it is necessary to further describe which energy system might be more affected. An instrument that might offer valuable information, whether the exercise limitation is more anaerobic or more aerobic in nature, is the calculation of the ratio of anaerobic to aerobic power (Blimkie et al., 1986). The objective of this study was to examine the aerobic-to-anaerobic power ratio in children with JIA compared with healthy peers.

29.2   METHODS

Sixty-two children with JIA (mean ± SD age 11.9 ± 2.1 years, range 7.2-15.9 years) with varying severity of disease participated in this study. The patients were diagnosed with JIA according to the International League of Associations for Rheumatology criteria. During the tests, 35 patients had active disease, 12 patients were in clinical remission and taking medication, and 15 patients were in clinical remission and off medication. All the tests and measurements of the patients were performed on the same day, with enough resting time between the anaerobic and aerobic exercise tests. The anaerobic test was always performed first. The outcome values of the measurements of the patients with JIA were compared with age-, weight-, and sex-matched reference values obtained from 50 healthy Dutch children, as reported previously (Van Leeuwen et al., 2004). Informed consent was obtained from the parents and/or from the children if they were <12 years of age. The Medical Ethics Committee of the University Medical Center Utrecht approved all study procedures.

Before the abovementioned exercise tests began, the anthropometry (body mass, height, BMI, and subcutaneous adiposity), joint status (number of tender and swollen joints), joint mobility (pEPMROM), and functional ability (CHAQ) of every participating child was determined. The Wingate Anaerobic Test (WAnT) during a 30 sec all-out cycle ergometer test and the maximal oxygen uptake ($\dot{V}O_{2peak}$) attained during a graded maximal exercise test to volitional exhaustion were both performed on a calibrated electromagnetic braked cycle ergometer (Lode Examiner; Lode, Groningen, The Netherlands). Material and methods of both exercise tests were as reported previously (Van Brussel et al., 2007). During the WAnT, external resistance was controlled, the power output was measured, and mean mechanical anaerobic power (MAnP) and peak mechanical anaerobic power (PAnP) were calculated from the exercise results. The highest achieved power output during the maximal exercise test was taken as the peak mechanical aerobic power (PAP). The anaerobic-to-aerobic power ratio was calculated as the ratio between the anaerobic mechanical power and aerobic mechanical power in watts. Statistical comparisons were made using linear regression. Differences between subgroups of JIA were tested using analysis of variance. P values less than 0.05 were considered significant.

29.3   RESULTS

All children were able to complete these tests without adverse effects. The differences between JIA patients and controls on MAnP, PAnP, and PAP were statistically significant ($P<0.05$). However, compared with healthy children, there were no significant differences in the mean anaerobic-to-aerobic power ratio or peak anaerobic-to-aerobic power ratios ($P= 0.52$ and $P= 0.99$, respectively). Moreover, there were no significant associations between mean anaerobic-to-aerobic power ratio, peak anaerobic-to aerobic power ratio, and CHAQ score (r = 0.2, r = 0.18, $P>0.05$), or pEPMROM score (r = 0.2, r = 0.22, $P>0.05$) even when adjusted for sex and/or age. Finally, there were no significant differences in mean anaerobic-to-aerobic power ratio and peak anaerobic-to-aerobic power ratio between girls and boys with JIA (*P*= 0.19 and *P*= 0.25, respectively), nor between healthy girls and boys (*P*= 0.08 and *P*= 0.09, respectively) (Figure 29.1a and 29.1b).

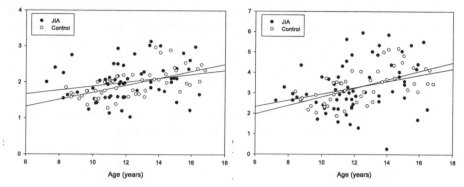

Figure. 29.1a (left panel) and **Figure 29.1b** (right panel): Development of mean and peak anaerobic-to-aerobic power ratio in children with JIA and healthy controls.

There were no statistically significant differences between JIA patients and healthy controls concerning mean anaerobic-to-aerobic power ratio and peak anaerobic-to-aerobic power ratio when corrected for age, height, and body mass due to overlap in 95%CIs. No statistically significant differences were observed in mean anaerobic-to-aerobic power ratio (F=0.21, *P*=0.81) and peak anaerobic-to-aerobic power ratio (F=0.51, *P*= 0.95) between the different disease-onset types of JIA. Development of the mean anaerobic-to-aerobic power ratio and peak anaerobic-to-aerobic power ratio in children with JIA and healthy controls in relation to age appears to be comparable (Van Brussel *et al.*, 2009).

29.4   DISCUSSION

We found that although both aerobic and anaerobic capacity were significantly reduced in the children with JIA, both mean anaerobic-to-aerobic power ratio and peak anaerobic-to-aerobic power ratios were no different between children with JIA and healthy controls. Moreover, there were no statistically significant differences between the subgroups of JIA in either mean anaerobic-to-aerobic power ratio or peak anaerobic-to-aerobic power ratio. We also confirmed a normal age-related increase in the power ratios in children with JIA. In the literature, peak anaerobic-to-aerobic power ratio is said to increase continuously from early childhood (Blimkie *et al.*, 1986). We found a similar increase in anaerobic-to-aerobic power ratio from early childhood in both children with JIA and healthy controls. There was no difference in the degree of the ratio change during growth between children with JIA and healthy controls, suggesting that the deficits in exercise tolerance affect aerobic and anaerobic capacity to a similar degree. This information is useful when defining rehabilitation or exercise training programs for this population. However, for a given age, there was a large range, more so than for healthy children, in power ratios between patients. We expect it is this individual variability that is important for the design of individualized exercise programs. Since the typical physical activity behaviour of healthy children (short bursts of intense activities separated by periods of rest) is anaerobic in nature (Bailey *et al.*, 1995), it is reasonable to expect that interventions focusing on anaerobic fitness of children with JIA may be of benefit. Although improvement of anaerobic power through exercise training has not been investigated in children with JIA, we have observed improvements in function and fitness with anaerobic exercise training in children with other chronic conditions. Given the apparently similar deficits in anaerobic capacity of youth with JIA, exercise training of the anaerobic energy system (e.g., high intensity interval training) might be equally valuable as the training of the aerobic system and, therefore, warranted in children with arthritis, especially those with a low anaerobic-to-aerobic power ratio.

29.5   REFERENCES

Bailey, R.C., Olson, J., Pepper, S.L., Porszasz, J., Barstow, T.J. and Cooper, D.M., 1995, The level and tempo of children's physical activities: an observational study. *Medicine and Science in Sports and Exercise*, **27**, pp. 1033–1041.

Blimkie, C.J., Roche, P. and Bar-Or, O., 1986, Anaerobic-to-aerobic power ratio in adolescent boys and girls. In: Rutenfranz J., Roche P., Bar-Or O., (Eds). *Children and exercise XII*. Champaign (IL): Human Kinetics, pp. 31–37.

Klepper, S.E., 2003, Exercise and fitness in children with arthritis: evidence of benefits for exercise and physical activity. *Arthritis and Rheumatism*, **49**, pp. 435–443.

Metin, G., Ozturk, L., Kasapcopur, O., Apelyan, M., and Arisoy, N., 2004, Cardiopulmonary exercise testing in juvenile idiopathic arthritis. *Journal of Rheumatology*, **31**, pp. 1834–1839.

Takken, T., Hemel, A., van der Net, J. and Helders, P.J., 2002, Aerobic fitness in children with juvenile idiopathic arthritis: a systematic review. *Journal of Rheumatology*, **29**, pp. 2643–2647.

Takken, T., van Brussel, M., Engelbert, R.H., van der Net, J., Kuis, W. and Helders, P.J., 2008, Exercise therapy in juvenile idiopathic arthritis: a Cochrane Review. *European Journal of Physical Rehabilitation Medicine*, **44**, pp. 287–297.

Van Brussel, M., Lelieveld, O.T., van der Net, J., Engelbert, R.H., Helders, P.J. and Takken, T., 2007, Aerobic and anaerobic exercise capacity in children with juvenile idiopathic arthritis. *Arthritis and Rheumatism*, **57**, pp. 891–897.

Van Brussel, M., van Doren, L., Timmons, B.W., Obeid, J., van der Net, J., Helders, P.J. and Takken, T., 2009, Anaerobic-to-aerobic power ratio in children with Juvenile Idiopathic Arthritis. *Arthritis and Rheumatism*, **61**, pp. 787–793

Van Leeuwen, P.B., van der Net, J., Helders, P.J. Takken, T., 2004, Exercise parameters in healthy Dutch children. *Geneeskunde en Sport*, **37**, pp. 126–132.

Aerobic Fitness and Performance Indices of Repeated Sprint Test in Normal Weight and Overweight Children

Y. Meckel[1], S. Lougassi[1], Y. Sitbon[1], D. Nemet[2], and A. Eliakim[1,2]

[1]Zinman College of Physical Education and Sport Sciences, Wingate Institute, Israel; [2]Child Health and Sport Center, Pediatric Department, Meir Medical Center, Sackler School of Medicine, Tel-Aviv University, Israel

30.1   INTRODUCTION

Previous studies have found that prepubescent boys needed less recovery time to sustain peak power output compared to pubescent boys and to young adults during repeated sprints (Ratel et al., 2006). It was also suggested that high level of aerobic fitness is a prerequisite for increased anaerobic performance during repeated sprints in adults (Taylor et al., 1997; Tomlin and Wenger, 2001). However, correlation analyses between $\dot{V}O_2$ max and performance indices of repeated sprint test (RST) have been inconsistent in this population (Meckel et al., 2009). These relationships were never studied in normal weight and overweight children. Therefore, the aim of the present study was to determine the relationship between RST (i.e., 12 x 20 m) and aerobic fitness (measured by the distance completed during 20 m shuttle run test) in pre- and early-pubertal normal weight and overweight children.

30.2   METHODS

30.2.1 Procedure

Eighteen normal weigh (35.9±6.3 kg), and fourteen overweight (52.5±10.0 kg) children (10.3±1.5 yrs) performed two tests:

a) Aerobic power test - Twenty-Meter Shuttle Run Test. The test consisted of shuttle running at increasing speeds between two markers placed 20 m apart. A portable compact disc (Sony CFD-V7) dictated the pace of the test by emitting tones at appropriate intervals. A starting speed of 8.5 km/hour was maintained for one minute, and thereafter the speed was increased every minute by 0.5 km/hour. The test was terminated when the child withdrew voluntarily from the exercise, or failed to arrive within 3 meters of the end line on two consecutive tones. The aerobic fitness of each participant was calculated as the number of laps or total distance achieved during the test.

b) 12 X 20 m RST. The protocol consisted of 12 X 20 m runs starting every 20 seconds. A photoelectric cell timing system (Alge-Timing Electronic, Austria) linked to a digital chronoscope was used to record each sprint and rest interval time with an accuracy of 0.001 second. The three measures of the RST were the fastest 20 m sprint time (FS), the total sprint time (TS) of the 12 sprints, and the performance decrement (PD) during the test. Total sprint time was calculated as the sum of all sprints times of the test. Performance decrement was used as an indication of fatigue and was calculated as (TS/FS x 12 x 100) – 100 (Fitzsimons *et al.*, 1993).

Heart rate was measured using a Polar heart rate monitor (Polar Accurex Plus, Polar Electro, NY) immediately after completion of each run in the RST. Rate of perceived exertion (RPE) was determined using the modified Borg scale (Borg 1982) at the end of the RST.

30.2.2 Statistical analysis

A two-way repeated measure ANOVA with Bonferroni adjustments was used to compare differences (total distance 20 m shuttle run, RST's FS, TS, PD, heart rate, RPE) between the normal weight and overweight children. Pearson correlations were computed between the calculated distance during the shuttle run aerobic test and performance indices of the 12 x 20 m RST. Data are presented as mean ± SD.

30.3   RESULTS

Anthropometric characteristics, RST's performance indices and the results of the 20 m shuttle run aerobic test are presented in Table 30.1. Aerobic fitness, FS, and TS were significantly higher ($p<0.05$) in the normal weight compared to the overweight children. RPE was significantly lower in the normal weight children. Significant negative correlations (Figure 30.1) were found between aerobic fitness and TS (r= -0.802), FS (r= -0.762) and PD (r= -0.670) of the RST in normal weight children. Significant negative correlations were also found between aerobic fitness and TS (r= -0.767) and FS (r= -0.738) of the RST in overweight children.

Table 30.1. Anthropometric measures, RST performance indices and aerobic fitness of the normal and overweight children (Mean ± SD, * p<0.05, normal versus overweight).

Parameters	Normal weight (n=18)	Overweight (n=14)
Age (yrs)	10.4±1.2	10.6±1.5
Pubertal Stage (Tanner)	1.1±0.3	1.2±0.4
Body Height (m)	141.0±9.9	143.5±7.9
Body Weight (kg)	36.3±6.6	52.5±10.0*
BMI (kg/m^2)	18.1±1.5	25.1±4.7*
BMI Percentile (%)	59.8±12.9	96.4±1.9*
Fastest Sprint (sec)	4.10±0.34	4.71±0.65*
Total Sprint Time (sec)	52.99±4.95	60.03±9.05*
Performance Decrement (%)	7.74±3.55	6.36±3.62
Maximal Heart Rate (beats/min)	197.2±8.9	191.0±7.1
RPE Score	3.8±1.4	5.1±1.5*
Distance-20m Shuttle Run (m)	752.6±401.7	468.6±107.4*

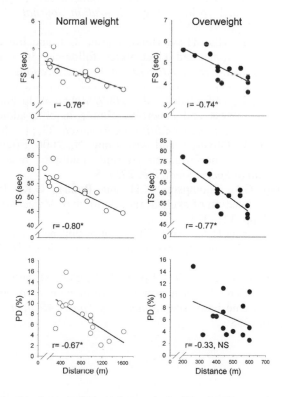

Figure 30.1. Relationships between the total distance in the 20 m shuttle run and performance indices of the RST in normal weight (left panel) and overweight (right panel) children. * p<0.05.

30.4   CONCLUSIONS

In pre-pubertal children the aerobic fitness and the anaerobic capabilities, of normal weight children are significantly higher than overweight children (Unnithan *et al.*, 2006). In addition, aerobic fitness plays an important role in intense intermittent activity in normal weight and overweight children. Finally, the results of the present study suggest that oxidative metabolism may serve as an energy source, even during a single sprint (Hebestreit *et al.*, 1996) in normal and in overweight children. Further studies are needed to clarify the relationships between the aerobic and the anaerobic capabilities in normal and overweight children and to observe the relative contribution of the aerobic and the anaerobic energy systems to short all-out exercise in pre- and early-pubertal children.

30.5   REFERENCES

Borg, G.A., 1982, Psychophysical bases of perceived exertion. *Medicine and Science in Sports and Exercise*, **14**, pp. 377–382.

Fitzsimons, M., Dawson, B.T., Ward, D. and Wilkinson, A., 1993, Cycling and running tests of repeated sprint ability. *Australian Journal of Science and Medicine in Sport*, **25**, pp. 82–87.

Hebestreit, H., Meyer, F., Htay-Htay, Heigenhauser, G.J. and Bar-Or, O., 1996, Plasma metabolites, volume and electrolytes following 30 s high-intensity exercise in boys and men. *Eurpean Journal of Applied Physiology*, **72**, pp. 563–569.

Meckel, Y., Machnai, O. and Eliakim, A., 2009, Relationship among repeated sprint tests, aerobic fitness and anaerobic fitness in elite adolescent soccer players. *Journal of Strength and Conditioning Research*, **23**, pp. 163–169.

Ratel, S., Williams, C.A., Oliver, J. and Armstrong, N., 2006, Effects of age and recovery duration on performance during multiple treadmill sprints. *International Journal of Sports Medicine*, **27**, 1–8.

Taylor, D.J., Kemp, G.J., Thompson, C.H. and Radda., G.K., 1997, Ageing: effects on oxidative function of skeletal muscle in vivo. *Molecular and Cellular Biochemestry*, **174**, pp. 321–324.

Tomlin, D.L. and Wenger, H.A., 2001, The relationship between aerobic fitness and recovery from high intensity intermittent exercise. *Sport Medicine*, **31**, pp. 1–11.

Unnithan, V.B., Nevill, A., Lange, G., Eppel, J., Fischer, M. and Hebestreit, H., 2006, Applicability of an allometric power equation to children, adolescents and young adults of extreme body size. *Journal of Sports Medicine and Physical Fitness*, **46**, pp. 202–208.

Aerobic Capacity in Contemporary Children and Adolescents with Cerebral Palsy

O. Verschuren[1], and T. Takken[2]

[1] Centre of Excellence, Rehabilitation Centre 'De Hoogstraat', Utrecht, The Netherlands; [2] Child Development & Exercise Center, Wilhelmina Children's Hospital, University Medical Centre Utrecht, Utrecht, The Netherlands

31.1 INTRODUCTION

To date, only four studies (Rieckert *et al.*, 1977; Lundberg, 1984; Hoofwijk *et al.*, 1995; Maltais *et al.*, 2005) have studied the $\dot{V}O_{2peak}$ in children and adolescents with cerebral palsy (CP) during a maximal exercise test. The most functional and appropriate way to assess the $\dot{V}O_{2peak}$ in children with CP who are able to walk independently, is a progressive walking or running-based maximal exercise test (Verschuren *et al.*, 2006). From three studies there are data available on $\dot{V}O_{2peak}$ in children with CP, which are based on a maximal exercise test on a treadmill (Rieckert *et al.*, 1977; Hoofwijk *et al.*, 1995; Maltais *et al.*, 2005). Hoofwijk *et al.* (1995) included 9 children with CP and compared the $\dot{V}O_{2peak}$ to the values in typically developing children and adolescents. The studies performed by Rieckert *et al.* (1977) and Maltais *et al.* (2005), examining respectively 12 and 11 children with CP, did not compare the results with typically developing children, but provided useful information on $\dot{V}O_{2peak}$ values for children with CP.

The current available data on $\dot{V}O_{2peak}$ in children with CP might be obsolete due to changing intervention programs for children and adolescents with CP (Damiano, 2006). Therefore, the purpose of this article is to describe the $\dot{V}O_{2peak}$ in contemporary children and adolescents with CP who are able to walk independently, using a maximal treadmill protocol, with the results being compared with normative values for age and gender. These results will be compared with the findings of earlier studies that assessed $\dot{V}O_{2peak}$ of children with CP using a maximal exercise test on a treadmill. Moreover, the differences between Gross Motor Functional Classification Scale (GMFCS) level I and II will be assessed as well.

31.2   METHODS

Twenty-four participants with CP (16 boys, 8 girls), classified at GMFCS level I and II, participated in this study. The patient group was compared with reference values obtained in a large group of healthy control subjects who were recruited from regular schools in The Netherlands. All participants performed a progressive treadmill exercise test to exhaustion (Binkhorst *et al.*, 1992). The healthy reference group was matched with the children and adolescents with CP according to age and gender. Physical characteristics of the patient group (according to GMFCS level) are summarized in Table 31.1. There were no significant differences between the groups.

Table 31.1. Subject characteristics.

	GMFCS Level I (n=13)			GMFCS Level II (n=11)		
Variable	Mean	SD	Range	Mean	SD	Range
Age (y)	11.2	2.8	7.5-16.1	12.5	3.0	7.2-17.0
Height (cm)	148.1	15.8	125-175	148.6	18.9	123-175
Body mass (kg)	39.4	11.6	23.8-60.8	38.6	12.1	24.0-59.7
Skin folds (mm)	34.4	14.4	20.5-69.0	36.0	10.6	22.5-60.0
Body mass index	17.7	3.6	14.2-26.1	17.7	2.3	13.9-21.4

GMFCS=Gross Motor Function Classification System.

To control for changes in body size during growth the $\dot{V}O_{2peak}$ (l/min) data were expressed as $\dot{V}O_{2peak}$/kg (ml/kg/min), and compared to reference values from age- and gender-matched Dutch controls (Binkhorst *et al.*, 1992). The $\dot{V}O_{2peak}$/kg values calculated for the subjects with CP were compared with $\dot{V}O_{2peak}$/kg values from previously published studies that performed a maximal exercise test on a treadmill (Rieckert *et al.*, 1977; Hoofwijk *et al.*, 1995; Maltais *et al.*, 2005). Based on the description of the subjects included in these three previously published studies the subjects have been classified according to the GMFCS levels.

Statistical comparisons between children and adolescents with CP and reference values were tested using a paired samples T-test. Differences between subgroups (GMFCS I and GMFCS II; boys and girls) were tested using an independent samples T-test ($\alpha = 0.05$).

31.3   RESULTS

$\dot{V}O_{2peak}$/kg of boys with CP was significantly lower (44.7 ± 7.1 ml/kg/min) than that of typically developing controls (51.7 ±1.2 ml/kg/min). There was also a significant difference between the girls with CP (36.4 ±7.6 ml/kg/min) and their typically developing controls (44.7 ± 0.3 ml/kg/min). There was no significant difference in $\dot{V}O_{2peak}$/kg between boys classified at GMFCS level I (44.6 ±6.3 ml/kg/min) and GMFCS level II (45.1 ±9.0 ml/kg/min). The $\dot{V}O_{2peak}$/kg among girls classified at GMFCS level I and GMFCS level II was not significantly different as well, 41.0 (±7.8 ml/kg/min) and 33.6 (±6.7 ml/kg/min) respectively (P>0.05).

Table 31.2 summarizes the findings on $\dot{V}O_{2peak}$/kg values in children and adolescents with CP who performed a maximal exercise test on a treadmill. The values found by Rieckert *et al.* (1977), Maltais *et al.* (2005) and Hoofwijk *et al.* (1995) are significantly lower than the present values.

Table 31.2. Survey of studies using $\dot{V}O_{2peak}$ testing in children with CP using a progressive exercise test on a treadmill.

Reference	No. of participants	Type of CP	GMFCS level	Age	$\dot{V}O_{2peak}$/kg (ml/kg/min)
Rieckert *et al.* (1977)	6 (1 boy and 5 girls)	3 quadriplegia 3 diplegia	III	7-19	28
	6 (4 boys and 2 girls)	4 hemiplegia 2 quadriplegia	I or II	14-18	34.7
Hoofwijk *et al.* (1995)	9 (7 boys, 2 girls)	1 hemiplegia 7 diplegia 1 quadriplegia	I or II	10-16	32.7
Maltais *et al.* (2005)	11 (7 boys, 4 girls)	7 hemiplegia 4 diplegia	I or II	10-16	34.0
Current study	24 (16 boys, 8 girls)	12 hemiplegia 12 diplegia	I or II	7-17	42.0

CP Cerbral Palsy; GMFCS=Gross Motor Function Classification System

31.4   DISCUSSION

The aerobic capacity of contemporary children and adolescents with CP, who are classified at GMFCS level I or II is significantly lower than that of typically developing controls. Furthermore, there was no significant difference in $\dot{V}O_{2peak}$ (ml/kg/min) between children and adolescents with CP, classified at GMFCS level I or II. However, the aerobic capacity in the subjects with CP from the current study reported higher values compared to values previously reported in the literature.

Traditional treatment of CP has focused primarily on attempting to improve abnormal motor patterns and maintain muscle length for daily activity and positioning. Theoretical shifts and research knowledge in the last two decades have encouraged therapists to consider interventions focusing on improving the aerobic capacity in children with CP (Damiano, 2006; Verschuren *et al.*, 2008). We therefore think that the higher $\dot{V}O_{2peak}$ values observed in the current study compared to previously published values reflect the change in treatment focus.

A recently published fitness program shows that a fitness training program with an aerobic and anaerobic training focus is able to improve the aerobic and anaerobic performance in children with CP, who are classified at GMFCS level I and II (Verschuren *et al.*, 2007). After this training program, observed improvements were 38% (2 sessions a week for 8 months) for aerobic performance estimated from a shuttle run test performance. Although long-term effects of fitness training are not known, one can only assume that an early introduction to a lifestyle that includes fitness would be beneficial for future health and function for children with CP. Physical therapists might consider fitness programs for children and adolescents with spastic CP by familiarizing them with exercising at school or in the community. Lifelong fitness habits formed at a young age begin with experience, success and satisfaction derived from the benefits of a good exercise program.

31.5   REFERENCES

Binkhorst, R.A., Hof van het, M.A. and Saris, W.H., 1992, *Maximum exercise in children; reference-values for 6-18 years old girls and boys*. Dutch Heart Association, The Hague, The Netherlands.

Damiano, D.L., 2006, Activity, Activity, Activity: Rethinking Our Physical Therapy Approach to Cerebral Palsy. *Physical Therapy*, **86**, pp. 1534–1540.

Hoofwijk, M., Unnithan, V.B. and Bar-Or, O., 1995, Maximal Treadmill Performance of Children with Cerebral Palsy. *Pediatric Exercise Science*, **7**, pp. 305–313.

Lundberg, A., 1984, Longitudinal study of physical working capacity of young people with spastic cerebral palsy. *Developmental Medicine and Child Neurology*, **26**, pp. 328–334.

Maltais, D., Pierrynowski, M., Galea, V. and Bar-Or, O., 2005, Physical Activity level is associated with the O_2 Cost of Walking in Cerebral Palsy. *Medicine and Science in Sports Exercise*, **37**, pp. 347–353.

Rieckert, H., Bruhm, U. and Schwalm, U., 1977, Endurance training within a program of physical education in children predominantly with cerebral palsy. *Medizinische Welt*, **28**, pp. 1694–1701.

Verschuren, O., Ketelaar, M., Gorter, J.W., Helders, P.J.M., Uiterwaal, C.S.P.M. and Takken, T., 2007, Exercise training program in children and adolescents with cerebral palsy: A randomized controlled trial. *Archives of Pediatrics and Adolescent Medicine*, **161**, pp. 1075–1081.

Verschuren, O., Ketelaar, M., Takken, T., Helders, P.J. and Gorter, J.W. , 2008, Exercise programs for children with cerebral palsy: a systematic review of the literature. *American Journal of Physical Medicine and Rehabilitation*, **87**, pp. 404–417.

Verschuren, O., Takken, T., Ketelaar, M., Gorter, J.W. and Helders, P.J.M., 2006, Reliability and Validity of Data for 2 Newly Developed Shuttle Run Tests in Children With Cerebral Palsy. *Physical Therapy*, **86**, pp. 1107–1117.

Physiological and Perceptual Responses in Children During Variable-Intensity Exercise

A.D. Mahon, L.M. Guth, and K.A. Craft

Human Performance Laboratory, Ball State University, Muncie, USA

32.1 INTRODUCTION

The study of exercise responses in children can be accomplished using any one of a number of well-established exercise testing protocols in the laboratory. For example, threshold responses and peak aerobic exercise capacity can be assessed using a graded exercise test (Mahon *et al.*, 2003). Anaerobic power is often assessed using the Wingate Anaerobic Test (Van Praagh and Doré, 2002). Constant work, submaximal exercise, is used to examine locomotion economy (Morgan *et al.*, 2004) or fuel use patterns (Stephens *et al.*, 2006). The assessment of oxygen uptake kinetic responses at the onset of submaximal exercise has been shown to be a viable non-invasive determinant of muscle oxidative capacity (Armstrong and Barker, 2009). Finally, repeated bouts of intense exercise performed for a fixed duration and rest interval have been used to assess characteristics of fatigue (Ratel *et al.*, 2006).

Variable-intensity exercise (VIE) is another form of exercise that can be performed in the laboratory setting. This type of exercise is characterized by frequent changes in a wide range of exercise intensities usually performed for relatively short periods of time and then repeated for a fixed amount of time. Recent examples of the use of a VIE protocol are the soccer-specific exercise protocol developed by Oliver *et al.* (2007) and the Loughborough Intermittent Shuttle Test (Nicholas *et al.*, 2000). Given the limited amount of research on exercise responses during VIE, especially in children, this study sought to evaluate the physiological and perceptual responses in children during VIE with particular regard to the day-to-day consistency in these responses. The specific aim of the study was to determine the suitability of a standard VIE protocol that could be used in future studies assessing fatigue, exercise performance, energy metabolism and supplementation.

32.2 METHODS

Six children (5 girls and 1 boy) with a mean (± SD) age of 12.8 ± 2.1 yrs, stature of 157.0 ± 11.1 cm, and mass of 53.7 ± 16.4 kg served as subjects in this study. Prior to participation parent permission and child assent were given in accordance with Institutional Review Board requirements. The children were required to report to the laboratory on four separate days. The first day served as a familiarization and orientation session; on the second visit, a graded exercise test was performed to determine peak aerobic exercise responses; and, on the final two visits, the children performed the VIE protocol in an identical manner on each day.

During the first visit, the child's stature and mass were recorded and he or she was oriented to the use of a rating of perceived exertion (RPE) scale. The child then performed a graded exercise test on a cycle ergometer to a near peak effort. During this bout a mouthpiece breathing valve and nose clip were used to measure pulmonary gas exchange; heart rate (HR) was recorded at 30-second intervals; and, RPE was assessed at the end of exercise test stage. Following a 15-minute rest period, one 12-minute set of the VIE protocol that would be used during the third and fourth visits was performed. During the VIE protocol HR and RPE were recorded at six and 12 minutes.

On a second day, a graded exercise test was performed to determine peak aerobic work capacity. The protocol began at 25 or 50 W for 2 minutes and increased by 25 W/2 minutes until a near peak effort was attained. Thereafter, further increases in power output occurred at 12 or 13 W/minute until peak voluntary effort was achieved. Pulmonary gas exchange was assessed continuously. HR was recorded at 30-second intervals and RPE was recorded at the end of each test stage. In order to ascertain that a peak effort was achieved, two of the following four criteria were required to be apparent: respiratory exchange ratio ≥ 1.00/1.05 depending on the child's age, HR ≥ 95% of age-predicted maximum (Tanaka *et al.*, 2001), a pedal rate < 50 rpm's, and/or an RPE ≥ 8. Criteria attainment ranged from two to four. Peak exercise responses for $\dot{V}O_2$, HR, RER, RPE and power output were recorded. Power output was prorated relative to the duration of the final exercise test stage.

The VIE protocol was performed on the third and fourth days and consisted of three sets of exercise each performed for 12 minutes with a three to four minute rest period interspersed between sets. A five-minute warm-up period preceded the first set. Each set of exercise consisted of six repeating cycles performed at a percentage of peak aerobic power output capacity as follows: 20 seconds at 25%, 30 seconds at 50%, 20 seconds at 125%, 30 seconds at 25%, and 20 seconds at 75%. HR and RPE were recorded at the sixth and twelfth minute of each set. Pulmonary gas exchange was measured throughout the second set of exercise and averaged in two-minute segments over the last 10 minutes of the set. Capillary blood samples were obtained prior to exercise, during the rest periods, and at the end of the protocol. For each child the VIE trials were performed at approximately the same time of day, and the children were instructed to refrain from vigorous activity and caffeine intake on the day of testing. Food intake was restricted in the three to four hours prior to testing.

All exercise testing was performed on a Lode Excalibur cycle ergometer. Pulmonary gas exchange was measured using standard open circuit spirometry gas exchange methods. HR was assessed with a Polar heart monitor, and RPE was determined using the OMNI cycle RPE scale (Robertson *et al.*, 2000). Glucose was analyzed using an automated device and lactate was determined using a standard enzymatic assay (Passonneau and Lowry, 1993).

Descriptive statistics (M ± SD) are presented for peak exercise responses. A two-way (day x time) ANOVA was used to analyze for the exercise responses during the VIE trials. Where appropriate, significant findings were further analyzed using a Bonferroni *post-hoc* test. Intra-class correlation coefficients calculated for paired responses across day. Statistical significance set to $p < 0.05$.

32.3 RESULTS

At peak exercise, oxygen uptake ($\dot{V}O_2$) was 1.89 ± 0.29 L/min and 36.8 ± 7.1 ml/kg/min. HR averaged 186 ± 16 bpm, RER was 1.17 ± 0.06, and RPE was 7.8 ± 1.7 at this level of exertion and power output averaged 159 ± 40 W.

The pulmonary gas exchange responses during the second set of exercise are outlined in Table 32.1. The day, time and the interaction effects for $\dot{V}O_2$ were not significant. When expressed as percentage of peak $\dot{V}O_2$, the average exercise intensity during the VIE trials ranged from 70% to 75%. Similar to $\dot{V}O_2$, there were no significant findings with this variable. In contrast, pulmonary ventilation ($\dot{V}_E$) increased over time ($p < 0.05$). Specifically, the $\dot{V}_E$ at 4 minutes was less than the values at 8 and 12 minutes. There were no day or interaction effects for this variable. The intra-class correlations for all comparisons were significant for both $\dot{V}O_2$ and $\dot{V}_E$.

Table 32.1. Pulmonary gas exchange responses during the second set of VIE (n = 5).

Variable	Day	Time (min)				
		4	6	8	10	12
$\dot{V}O_2$	1	1.34±0.28	1.32±0.31	1.37±0.29	1.39±0.28	1.34±0.23
(L/min)						
	2	1.36±0.28	1.39±0.29	1.38±0.29	1.36±0.31	1.41±0.30
ICC		0.99	0.93	0.98	0.99	0.92
$\dot{V}_E$	1	40.8±10.8	42.3±11.5	44.1±10.5	44.7±9.1	44.4±8.5
(L/min)						
	2	40.2±9.5	44.1±10.0	44.8±10.9	43.1±11.7	46.2±11.5
ICC		0.99	0.93	0.90	0.91	0.83

ICC = intra-class correlation; $\dot{V}_E$ = pulmonary ventilation

The blood lactate and glucose concentrations during the VIE on each day are shown in Table 32.2. There was no day or interaction effect for lactate concentration. However, lactate concentration increased with all three exercise values significantly higher than pre-exercise. There were no significant effects for glucose concentration. All of the intra-class correlations for the lactate comparisons were significant; however, only the pre-exercise and 12-minute intra-class correlations were significant for the glucose comparisons.

Table 32.2. Blood lactate and glucose concentration during VIE across two days.

Variable	Day	Time (min)			
		Pre	12	24	36
Lactate (mmol/L)	1	1.3±0.3	5.7±1.9	5.3±2.0	5.1±1.9
	2	1.4±0.3	5.1±2.0	5.2±1.9	4.8±2.0
ICC		0.60	0.86	0.89	0.85
Glucose (mmol/L)	1	98.3±8.2	91.0±18.0	97.0±5.7	93.0±13.5
	2	97.0±10.5	97.2±12.5	90.8±6.4	89.3±9.9
ICC		0.79	0.70	0.23	0.33

ICC = intra-class correlation

The HR and RPE responses during each VIE are shown in Figures 32.1 and 32.2, respectively. For HR there was no difference between days of testing, nor was there an interaction. However, across time there were significant differences in HR. Specifically, HR at 6 minutes was lower versus 12 minutes and 24 minutes and the HR at 30 minutes was lower than at 36 minutes. Similar results were apparent for RPE, that is the day and interaction effects were not significant, while the time effect was significant. However, *post-hoc* testing on the time effect revealed only one pairwise difference between the RPE at minute 18 versus the RPE at minute 36. The intra-class correlations for HR were all in excess or 0.90 (p < 0.05), however for RPE, only the first two pairwise comparisons were significantly related (r = 0.85), while the other four comparisons were not significant and ranged from r = 0.11 to 0.60.

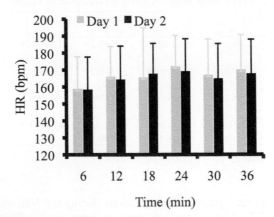

Figure 32.1. Heart rate (HR) response during each variable-intensity.

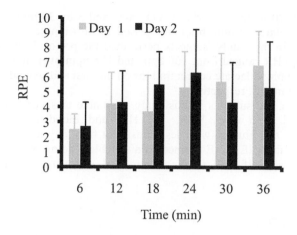

Figure 32.2. Rating of perceived exertion (RPE) response during each variable-intensity.

32.4 DISCUSSION

This study examined the physiological and perceptual responses to VIE. The results indicated that measures of gas exchange, specifically $\dot{V}O_2$ and $\dot{V}_E$ along with HR and blood lactate concentration were quite reproducible across two different days of exercise. Less reproducible were measures of blood glucose and RPE. Blood glucose reproducibility may have been compromised by the fact that the children did not perform the VIE each day under tightly controlled nutritional conditions. The children were instructed to report to the laboratory several hours from their last meal and attempt to eat a similar diet each day, but variations may have confounded the results. RPE also showed poor day-to-day reliability. However, examination of the individual responses indicates much of the inability to reproduce the RPE could be attributed to one subject who demonstrated much variation within and between days for his RPE selections. Removal of this one subject from the data analysis increase the ICCs to > 0.78.

There have been several recent studies which have examined VIE responses in children and adults. Oliver *et al.* (2007) developed a soccer-specific protocol which required adolescent boys to walk, jog and sprint on a non-motorized treadmill in the following manner: 45 seconds at 4 km/hr, 15 seconds at 12 km/hr, 15 seconds standing, 40 seconds at 8 km/hr, and 5 seconds of maximal sprinting. This two-minute cycle was then repeated seven times for a set; the set was then repeated two more times. Similar to the present study, the average intensity was ~70% of peak $\dot{V}O_2$ over the final two sets. The average HR during all three sets ranged from 173 to 176 bpm which is also very similar to the responses observed in this study; the blood lactate concentrations ranged from 7.2 mmol/L at the end of the first set to 6.9 mmol/L following the third set. The Loughborough Intermittent Shuttle Test, developed using adult subjects, is another type of VIE protocol that has appeared in the literature (Nicholas *et al.*, 2000). This protocol consists of a series of 20-meter segments as follows over a 15 minute period of time: 3 by 20 meters walking, 3 by 20 meters running at maximal speed, 4 seconds of recovery, 3 by 20 meters at 55% of $\dot{V}O_2$max, and 3 by 20 meters at 95 % of $\dot{V}O_2$max. After a three-minute brief rest period the 15-minute set was repeated four more times. In this study, subjects performed the protocol on two different days. The average HR ranged from 166 bpm and 178 bpm over time and between days. The average blood lactate concentrations on the first and second day were 5.7 mmol/L and 6.2 mmol/L, respectively.

In conclusion, the subjects in this study were able to successfully complete the VIE protocol each day. $\dot{V}O_2$, $\dot{V}_E$, HR, and blood lactate were very reproducible. RPE and glucose were less consistent from day to day especially in the later stages of the VIE. VIE protocol is a suitable type of exercise to study in children and lends itself well to the intermittent and varied nature of sports participation

32.5   REFERENCES

Armstrong, N. and Barker, A.R., 2009, Oxygen uptake kinetics in children and adolescents: a review. *Pediatric Exercise Science*, **21**, pp. 130–147.

Mahon, A.D., Plank, D.M. and Hipp, M.J., 2003, The influence of exercise test protocol on perceived exertion at submaximal exercise intensities in children. *Canadian Journal of Applied Physiology*, **28**, pp. 53–63.

Morgan, D.W., Tseh, W., Caputo, J.L., Keefer, D.J., Craig, I.S., Griffith, K.B., Akins, M.B., Griffith, G.E., Krahenbuhl, G.S. and Martin, P.E., 2004, Longitudinal stratification of gait economy in young boys and girls: the locomotion energy and growth study. *European Journal of Applied Physiology*, **91**, pp. 30–34.

Nicholas, C.W., Nuttall, F.E. and Williams, C., 2000, The Loughborough Intermittent Shuttle Test: a field test that simulates the activity pattern of soccer. *Journal of Sports Sciences*, **18**, pp. 97–104.

Oliver, J.L., Armstrong, N. and Williams, C.A., 2007, Reliability and validity of a soccer-specific test of prolonged repeated-sprint ability. *International Journal of Sports Physiology and Performance*, **2**, pp. 137–149.

Passonneau, J.V. and Lowry, O.H., 1993, *Enzymatic Analysis: A Practical Guide*, (Totowa, NJ: Humana Press).

Ratel, S., Williams, C.A., Oliver, J. and Armstrong, N., 2006, Effects of age and recovery duration on performance during multiple treadmill sprints. *International Journal of Sports Medicine*, **27**, pp. 1–8.

Robertson, R.J., Goss, F.L., Boer, N.F., Peoples, J.A., Foreman, A.J., Dabayebeh, I.M., Millich, N.B., Balaskaran, G., Riechman, S.E., Gallagher, J.D. and Thompkins, T., 2000, Children's OMNI scale of perceived exertion: mixed gender and race validation. *Medicine and Science in Sports and Exercise*, **32**, pp. 452–458.

Stephens, B.R., Cole, A.S. and Mahon, A.D., 2006, The influence of biological maturation on fat and carbohydrate metabolism during exercise in males. *International Journal of Sport Nutrition and Exercise Metabolism*, **16**, pp. 166–179.

Tanaka, H., Monahan, K.D. and Seals, D.R., 2001, Age-predicted maximal heart rate revisited. *Journal of the American College of Cardiology*, **37**, pp. 153–156.

Van Praagh, E. and Doré, E., 2002, Short-term muscle power during growth and maturation. *Sports Medicine*, **32**, pp. 701–728.

Part VI

Fitness Assessment

Assessment of Anaerobic Performance in Youth Basketball and its Contribution to Differentiate Players by Competitive Level

M.J. Coelho e Silva[1], H. Moreira Carvalho[1], A.M.C. Santos[1], C.E. Gonçalves[1], A.J. Figueiredo[1], M. Mazzuco[2], and R.M. Malina[3-4]

[1]Faculty of Sport Science and Physical Education, University of Coimbra, Portugal; [2]Federal University of Paraná, Brazil; [3]Professor Emeritus, Department of Kinesiology and Health Education, University of Texas, Austin, USA; [4]Research Professor, Department of Health and Physical Education, Tarleton State University, Stephenville, Texas, USA

33.1 INTRODUCTION

Regeneration of muscle ATP through nonoxidative mechanisms is an essential feature in training and performance. Efforts of short duration and maximum intensity often occur during basketball games and frequently during decisive moments (Ben Abdelkrim *et al.*, 2007; McInnes *et al.*, 1995). It is generally accepted that anaerobic energy production mechanisms are important features of talent development programs and sport-specific fitness testing (Pearson *et al.*, 2006), but relatively little information is available on the contribution of anaerobic metabolism to success in young athletes, including basketball players. Moreover, the value of testing is frequently debated in the context of the relative accuracy of field versus laboratory protocols. Although laboratory tests are performed under controlled conditions, motivation is generally higher in conditions that approximate game situations (Van Praagh and França, 1998). The present study had two objectives (1) to evaluate associations between the Wingate [WanT] laboratory test and two field protocols [140-m line drill, 7-sprints] of anaerobic performance, and (2) to test the efficacy of concurrent protocols to discriminate adolescent players by competitive level.

33.2   METHODS

The sample included 55 adolescent basketball players (15.2±0.6 years). Stature, weight and dimensions needed to estimate total and fat-free thigh volumes (TLV, FFLV) were measured (Jones and Pearson, 1969). Anaerobic assessments were done on three occasions with three protocols: 30-s WanT (Bar-Or, 1987), 7-sprint test (Bangsbo, 1994) and the 140-m line drill (Apostolidis et al., 2004; Hoffman et al., 1999). After a warm-up, the subject performed 7 sprints of about 35 m each. The protocol provides the faster of the first two sprints, the slower of the last two sprints, and the sum of the 7 sprints (Bangsbo, 1994). The 140-m shuttle run required the subject to perform 140 m as fast as possible in four consecutive shuttle sprints of 5.8, 14.0, 22.2 and 28.0 m on an official basketball court (Seminick, 1990). Time was recorded using a photoelectric cell apparatus (Globus Ergo Timer Timing System, Codogné, Italy). The WAnT test used a Monark cycle ergometer (model 824E) coupled with a *Baumer sensor* (model CH-8500 Frauenfeld). The warm-up consisted of pedalling at 60 rpm for 4 minutes, interspersed with a sprint of 3 to 5 seconds against a resistance of 7.5% of body mass at the end of the 1st, 2nd and 3rd minutes. The following were derived: anaerobic peak power (APP) which corresponds the ability to produce short-term mechanical power; anaerobic mean power (AMP) which reflects intermediate-term performance (Bar-Or, 1987 ; Martin and Malina, 1998); and also the fatigue index. Based on the outputs, it was possible to derive absolute (W) and relative anaerobic performance ($W.kg^{-1}$, by unit of body mass; $W.L^{-1}$, by unit of thigh volume). The correlations among tests were calculated. Subsequently, analyses of variance (ANOVA) and covariance (ANCOVA, controlling for height, weight and thigh volume) were used to evaluate the effect of competitive level (local, elite) on the anaerobic indicators. The level of significance was set at 5%.

33.3   RESULTS

Correlations between field and laboratory assessments of anaerobic performance are summarized in Table 33.1. Correlations between the run tests and anaerobic peak and mean power were consistently higher when expressed per unit of body mass than per unit of thigh volume. Correlations were lower when anaerobic power was expressed in absolute values (watts). Correlations between sprint times and anaerobic peak power ($watts.kg^{-1}$) ranged from 0.55 (trial 7) and 0.61 (trial 1). The 140-m line drill was moderately correlated with relative values of peak and mean power (0.73-0.72, when expressed in $watts.kg^{-1}$; 0.59-0.60, when expressed in $watts.L^{-1}$). The fatigue indexes derived from the 7-sprint and WAnT protocols were not related to each other.

Table 33.1. Correlations between the Wingate and field tests (n=55).

7-sprint	Anaerobic peak power			Anaerobic mean power			FI
	W	W/kg^{-1}	W.L^{-1}	W	W.kg^{-1}	W.L^{-1}	
trial 1	0.38**	0.61**	0.49**	0.39**	0.59**	0.50**	-0.17
trial 2	0.29*	0.56**	0.41**	0.30*	0.56**	0.43**	-0.11
trial 3	0.34*	0.59**	0.47**	0.36**	0.60**	0.49**	-0.18
trial 4	0.37**	0.57**	0.51**	0.38**	0.56**	0.51**	-0.16
trial 5	0.36**	0.56**	0.50**	0.39**	0.58**	0.54**	-0.06
trial 6	0.37**	0.57**	0.49**	0.39**	0.58**	0.50**	-0.17
trial 7	0.32*	0.55**	0.46**	0.34*	0.56**	0.48**	-0.18
best trial	0.35**	0.62**	0.46**	0.36**	0.61**	0.46**	-0.20
sum	0.36**	0.60**	0.49**	0.38**	0.60**	0.51**	-0.15
fat. index	-0.13	-0.05	-0.24	-0.16	-0.11	-0.29*	0.03
140-SR	0.36**	0.73**	0.59**	0.37**	0.72**	0.60**	-0.27*

FI: Fatigue Index; 140-SR: 140-m shuttle run
* (p<0.05), ** (p<0.01). For time-scored events the signal was inverted because a lower time reflects a better performance.

Descriptive statistics for the local level and elite players are summarized in Table 33.2. The competitive groups differed significantly in height (F=32.47, p<0.01, h^2=0.38), weight (F=37.85, p<0.01, h^2=0.42) and thigh volume (TTV: F=11.28, p<0.01, h^2=0.18; FFTV: F=9.43, p<0.01, h^2=0.15). Elite players were taller (14.5 cm) and heavier (19.7 kg) and had a larger estimated thigh volume (0.56 L) than local level players. Local and elite players did not differ in the 7-sprint protocol when height, weight or thigh volume were statistically controlled (ANCOVA). Elite players were 1.31 s faster in the shuttle run test (F=4.82, p<0.05, h^2=0.08) and obtained higher outputs in anaerobic peak and mean power when expressed in watts (peak power: F=40.27, p<0.01, h^2=0.43; mean power: F=41.87, p<0.01, h^2=0.44) or watts . L^{-1} thigh volume (peak power: F=29.78, p<0.01, h^2=0.36; mean power: F=29.20, p<0.01, h^2=0.36), but not in W.kg^{-1}. The analysis of covariance (Table 33.3), controlling for height, showed significant differences between elite and local players only in anaerobic peak (F=6.64, p<0.01, h^2=0.11) and mean power (F=7.62, p<0.01, h^2=0.13). When body mass was the covariate, local and elite players were significantly differentiated by the 140-m shuttle run (F=6.64, p<0.01, h^2=0.11). When thigh volume was the covariate, the shuttle run (F=6.91, p<0.01, h^2=0.12), peak power (F=25.47, p<0.01, h^2=0.33) and mean power (F=25.71, p<0.01, h^2=0.34) significantly differentiated local and elite players.

Table 33.2. Descriptive statistics (mean±SD) and results of analyses of variance to test the effect of competitive level in anthropometry and anaerobic protocols.

	Local	Elite	F	p	η2
Height, cm	173.1±8.3	187.6±5.2	32.47	.00	.38
Weight, kg	63.0±9.8	82.7±9.8	37.85	.00	.42
Thigh total volume, L	4.28±0.52	4.84±0.45	11.28	.00	.18
Fat-free thigh volume; L	4.17±0.47	4.62±0.39	9.43	.00	.15
RSA: sprint 1, s	7.01±0.46	6.80±0.30	2.32	.13	.04
RSA: sprint 2, s	7.05±0.50	6.88±0.38	1.25	.27	.02
RSA: sprint 3, s	7.10±0.53	6.95±0.32	0.89	.35	.02
RSA: sprint 4, s	7.14±0.49	6.90±0.24	2.86	.10	.05
RSA: sprint 5, s	7.19±0.50	6.99±0.31	1.63	.21	.03
RSA: sprint 6, s	7.20±0.55	7.07±0.30	0.64	.43	.01
RSA: sprint 7, s	7.15±0.57	6.98±0.29	1.04	.31	.02
RSA: best sprint, s	6.97±0.48	6.77±0.29	1.89	.18	.03
RSA: sum of sprints, s	7.12±0.50	6.94±0.29	1.50	.23	.03
RSA: fatigue index, s	.312±0.27	0.32±0.14	0.00	.96	.00
140-m line drill, s	31.71±1.97	30.40±1.06	4.82	.03	.08
WanT: peak power, W	591.4±115.2	823.3±98.5	40.27	.00	.43
WanT: peak power, $W.kg^{-1}$	9.37±1.00	9.98±0.77	3.80	.06	.07
WanT: peak power, $W.L^{-1}$	137.8±19.6	170.1±10.65	29.78	.00	.36
WanT: mean power, W	508.0±93.4	702.1±85.9	41.87	.00	.44
WanT: mean power, $W.kg^{-1}$	8.06±0.84	8.52±0.81	2.88	.10	.05
WanT: peak power, $W.L^{-1}$	118.5±16.0	145.2±11.7	29.20	.00	.36
WanT: fatigue index	0.30±0.05	0.30±0.08	0.02	.88	.00

RSA: repeated sprint ability; 140-m run; WAnT: Wingate test

Table 33.3. Results of ANCOVA's controlling for the spurious effects of height (left), weight (middle) and thigh volume (right).

	covariate								
Variable,	Height			Weight			Thigh volume		
unit	F	p	η2	F	p	η2	F	p	η2
7-sprint test									
best trial, s	0.28	.60	.01	1.59	.21	.03	1.43	.24	.03
sum, s	0.00	.99	.00	0.70	.41	.01	1.16	.29	.02
fatigue index, s	3.74	.06	.07	1.04	.31	.02	0.00	.96	.00
140-m line drill, s	1.23	.27	.02	6.64	.01	.11	6.91	.01	.12
WanT									
peak power, W	6.64	.01	.11	2.97	.09	.05	25.47	.00	.33
mean power, W	7.62	.01	.13	3.82	.06	.07	26.71	.00	.34
fatigue index	0.04	.84	.00	0.03	.86	.00	0.01	.94	.00

33.4 DISCUSSION

Body mass and pubertal status have a significant influence on variation in power, aerobic endurance and sport-specific skills of basketball players 14-15 years (Coelho e Silva *et al.* , 2008). Since elite players were heavier than their local peers, which may be a consequence of earlier pubertal maturation, it was of interest to examine the contribution of anaerobic test protocols to the differentiation of players by competitive level statistically controlling for body size. With this approach, the 140-m run test appeared as the most informative protocol to distinguish players by competitive level when body weight was statistically controlled. This suggests that the test may be more sensitive to very intensive bouts of anaerobic capacity, which are perhaps more similar to those observed in match play. The WanT protocol requires the subject be in a seated position on the ergo-cycle, which may affect its specificity for basketball. In contrast, the repeated sprint protocol did not discriminate local and elite adolescent basketball players. Nevertheless, the three concurrent assessments of anaerobic performance showed substantial overlap in variance.

Documentation of the development of anaerobic performance in young athletes is relatively limited compared with an abundant literature describing the development of aerobic power. This may be due, in part, to the lack of valid and reliable testing protocols for assessing anaerobic power in young athletes. While protocols for anaerobic assessments are well established and validated in adults, their application to young athletes is less well established. Variation in pubertal status is a major confounder in physiological assessments of adolescent males. Variation in the timing and tempo of growth spurts in height and body mass may be an additional confounding factor. Age at peak height velocity, for example, precedes age at peak weight velocity so that there may be some dissociation of linear growth and muscular function at this time (Malina *et al.*, 2004).

Additional research is needed with adolescent basketball players. Results of the present study highlight the value of the 140 m shuttle protocol (line drill) in distinguishing players by competitive level. The concurrent test protocol may be of use in distinguishing athletes by playing position. Allometrically scaled anaerobic peak and mean power, and the addition of a force-velocity test should also be considered in future studies.

33.5 ACKNOWLEDGMENT

Fundação para Ciência e a Tecnologia [PTDC/DES/110159/2009]

33.6 REFERENCES

Apostolidis, N., Nassis, G.P., Bolatoglou, T. and Geladas, N.D., 2004, Physiological and technical characteristics of elite young basketball players. *Journal of Sports Medicine and Physical Fitness*, **44**, pp. 157–163.
Bangsbo, J., 1994., *Fitness Training in Football*. Bagsværd, Denmark, HO1Storm.

Bar-Or, O., 1987, The Wingate anaerobic test: an update on methodology, reliability and validity. *Sports Medicine*, **4**, pp. 381–391.

Ben Abdelkrim, N., El Fazaa, S. and El Ati, J., 2007, Time-motion analysis and physiological data of elite under-19-year-old basketball players during competition. *British Journal of Sports Medicine*, **41**, pp. 69–75.

Coelho e Silva, M. J., Figueiredo, A., Moreira Carvalho, H. and Malina, R.M., 2008, Functional capacities and sport-specific skills of 14-to 15-year-old male basketball players: size and maturity effects. *European Journal of Sport Science*, **8**, pp. 277–285.

Hoffman, J.R., Epstein, S., Einbinder, M. and Weinstein, Y., 1999, The Influence of Aerobic Capacity on Anaerobic Performance and Recovery Indices in Basketball Players. *Journal of Strength and Conditioning Research*, **13**, pp. 407–411.

Jones, P.R. and Pearson, J., 1969, Anthropometric determination of leg fat and muscle plus bone volumes in young male and female adults. *Journal of Physiology*, **204**, pp. 63–66.

Malina, R.M., Bouchard, C. and Bar-Or, O., 2004, *Growth, Maturation, and Physical Activity*. Champaign, IL: Human Kinetics.

Martin, J.C. and Malina, R.M., 1998, Developmental variations in anaerobic performance associated with age and sex. In E. V. Praagh (Ed.), *Pediatric Anaerobic Performance*, pp. 45–64. Champaign, IL: Human Kinetics.

McInnes, S.E., Carlson, J.S., Jones, C.J. and McKenna, M.J., 1995, The physiological load imposed on basketball players during competition. *Journal of Sports Science*, **13**, pp. 387–397.

Pearson, D.T., Naughton, G.A. and Torode, M., 2006, Predictability of physiological testing and the role of maturation in talent identification for adolescent team sports. *Journal of Science and Medicine in Sports*, **9**, pp. 277–287.

Seminick, D., 1990, Tests and measurements: The line drill test. *National Strength and Conditioning Athletic Journal*, **12**, pp. 47–49.

Van Praagh, E. and França, N., 1998, Measuring Maximal Short-Term Power Output During Growth. In E. V. Praagh (Ed.), *Pediatric Anaerobic Performance,* pp. 155–189. Champaign, IL: Human Kinetics.

Clinical Exercise Testing in Children with Neurometabolic Myopathies

T. Takken, C. Ernsting, H. Hulzebos, W.G. Groen, P. Van Hasselt, B. Prinsen, P.J.M. Helders, and G. Visser

Wilhelmina Children's Hospital, University Medical Center Utrecht, The Netherlands

34.1 INTRODUCTION

Although the value of exercise tests in neuromuscular disorders have been acknowledged for several decades (Brooke *et al.*, 1979; Carroll *et al.*, 1979; Sockolov *et al.*, 1977), the role of exercise as a diagnostic or therapeutic tool in children and adults with a metabolic myopathy (MM) and other neuromuscular disorders (NMD), has received less scientific attention compared to patients with heart and lung disease (Flaherty *et al.*, 2002; Haller and Lewis, 1984; Lewis and Haller, 1989).

Exercise testing can be used as a less invasive method to characterize patients with a suspected NMD and the results can be used for triage for further biochemical evaluations (Elliot *et al.*, 1989). Moreover, exercise tests can be helpful in prescribing safe but effective levels of physical activity (Devries and Tarnopolsky, 2008), or to evaluate the effect of exercise training or nutritional interventions for these patients (Taivassalo and Haller, 2004).

Therefore, the aim of the current study was to report the results of exercise tests in children with a diagnosed MM or other NMD. This information might be helpful for clinicians in the diagnosis and management of these disorders.

34.2 METHODS

Thirteen patients (9 boys, 4 girls, age 5-15 yrs) with a definite diagnosis of MM or NMD were included in this retrospective study. Their characteristics are displayed in Table 34.1. The results of nine children who were referred for exercise testing (3 girls, 6 boys, age: 12.3±3.8 years) in whom no diagnosis of an inherited MM or NMD could be made, were considered as the clinical control group for the biochemical measurements.

Cardiopulmonary exercise test (CPET) using cycle ergometry to determine the peak oxygen uptake ($\dot{V}O_{2peak}$) and peak work rate (W_{peak}) and a prolonged exercise test (PXT; 90-minutes at 30% of W_{peak}) were performed. During exercise respiratory gas-exchange and heart rate were monitored, and blood was drawn at set time points for biochemical analysis (e.g. CK, ammonia, lactate, acylcarnitine, FFA, and glucose). Urine was collected before exercise and during 3 hours after cessation of the test for examination (e.g. organic acids, purines, pyrimidines, and myoglobin). Methods were described in detail elsewhere (Takken *et al.*, 2005).

34.3   RESULTS

Results of the CPET are shown in Table 34.1. Patient 2 (GSD-III) stopped the CPET because of myalgia in the lower limbs.

$\dot{V}O_{2peak}$ and $\dot{V}O_{2peak}/kg$ were significantly reduced in several patients (3, 4, 10, 13). One patient with BMD (patient 12) had a high $\dot{V}O_{2peak}/kg$. Several patients (4 and 10) had to terminate the CPET because of muscular discomfort and exhaustion at a low HR_{peak}.

The patients with GSD-1a and mitochondrial myopathy (patient 1, and 10 respectively) had significantly increased lactate concentrations at rest, and one patient with BMD (patient 12) had an increased blood lactate concentration after the CPET. One patient with GSD-III and one with BMD (patients 2 and 12) had increased CK values at rest and after exercise. Ammonia concentrations were increased at rest in one patient with BMD (patient 12), and were reduced after the CPET in 2 patients (GSD-1a and mitochondrial myopathy).

Biochemical data of the PXT revealed that 3 patients, one with GSD-1a, GSD-7 and mitochondrial myopathy (patients 1, 3, 10 respectively) had an increased blood glucose concentration during exercise. Two patients, one with GSD-1a and the patients with mitochondrial myopathy (patients 1 and 10) showed significantly increased concentration of lactate at all time points. During and after exercise the CK value of the patient with GSD-7 (patient 3) was significantly increased. The two patients with BMD (patients 11, 12) had increased CK concentrations at rest as well as during exercise and recovery. Two patients, one with GSD-7 and one with BMD (patients 3 and 12 respectively) had significantly increased ammonia concentrations. There were no important significant differences in concentration of 3-keto-butyric acid and 3-OH-butyric acid between patients and the clinical control group.

Acylcarnitines C6, C8, C10, C12 and C14:1 were all increased in two patients with MADD (patients 7 and 8) in rest as well as during exercise. The patient with thiolase deficiency (patient 9) had increased C5:1 and C5-OH acylcarnitine during rest and exercise, as well as several increased organic acids in the urine. In the patient with mitochondrial myopathy (patient 10) C5 carnitine was increased.

Table 34.1. Characteristics of the patients and their peak results during cardio-pulmonary exercise testing.

#	Diagnosis	Determination of diagnosis	HR (bpm)	RER	$\dot{V}O_2$ (L/min) (Z-score)	$\dot{V}O_2$/kg (ml/min/kg) (Z-score)
1	GSD-1a	Mutation R570X en delta F327	205	1.16	1.99 (-0.04)	49.7 (-0.42)
2	GSD-III	Debranching enzyme deficiency in leucocytes	182	0.915	1.45 (-1.5)	37.1 (-1.5)
3	GSD-7	Phosphofructokinase deficiency in muscle	184	1.0	1.78 (-3.55)	34.6 (-3.24)
4	MCAD	MCAD deficiency in leucocytes homozygous Lys329Glu mutation	134	0.92	0.55 (-3.5)	19.5 (-4.2)
5	MCAD	MCAD deficiency in leucocytes	NA	NA	NA	NA
6	SCAD	SCAD deficiency in leucocytes and fibroblasts, mutation	173	1.05	1.00 (-0.86)	40.1 (-1.9)
7	MADD	MADD deficiency in fibroblasts	195	1.25	1.33 (-1.1)	40.4 (-1.8)
8	MADD	MADD deficiency in fibroblasts	180	1.21	1.29 (0.09)	51.5 (-0.26)
9	TD	2-Metylacetoacetyl-CoA-thiolase deficiency in fibroblasts	179	1.20	1.30 (-0.69)	43.5 (1.4)
10	MP	Diminished ATP production fresh muscle biopsy (respiratory chain defect)	152	1.39	0.63 (-3.6)	18.5 (-5.0)
11	BMD	Duplication exon 24-29 dystrophine gene	NA	NA	NA	NA
12	BMD	Duplication exon 24-29 dystrophine gene	202	1.26	1.57 (1.7)	62.6 (2.7)
13	HEP	Arg1239His mutation in CACNA1S-gene	218	1.25	1.20 (-2.0)	19.4 (-4.0)

GSD: glycogen storage disease, MCAD: Medium chain acyl CoA dehydrogenase deficiency, SCAD: short-chain acyl CoA dehydrogenase deficiency, MADD: Multiple Acyl CoA Dehydrogenase deficiency, TD: Thiolase deficiency, MM, Mitochondrial myopathy, BMD: Becker Muscular Dystrophy, HEP: Hypokalaemic episodic paralysis.

34.4   DISCUSSION

Because of the heterogeneity of the disorders, there was a large variation in the CPET and PXT results between patients. These differences reflect the different pathophysiology of the various disorders. In addition, this indicates that $\dot{V}O_{2peak}$ values are aspecific for a certain disorder. Patient 12 for example was a talented cyclist with a very high $\dot{V}O_{2peak}$ for his age. However during several races he developed myoglobinuria and he had quite high resting values of CK. Because his nephew was also referred with exercise intolerance to our hospital, an x-linked disorder was suspected. Muscle biopsies of the 2 boys revealed a duplication in exon 24-29 of the dystrophine gene, and the diagnosis of BMD was made. Based on these results the boy was advised to stop with high-level cycling.

Interpretation of the exercise test is not solely based on $\dot{V}O_{2peak}$ values; we also look for example at ventilatory threshold, oxygen uptake – work rate relationship, RER_{peak} and the appearance of metabolites in blood and urine.

In conclusion, CPET and PXT seem valuable instruments that can be of assistance in diagnosing patients with MD or NMD. Moreover exercise testing can help regarding the assessment of functional capacity in these patients and can give advice regarding safe and appropriate levels of physical activity and nutrition.

34.5   REFERENCES

Brooke, M.H., Carroll, J.E., Davis, J.E. and Hagberg, J.M., 1979, The prolonged exercise test. *Neurology*, **29**, pp. 636–643.

Carroll, J.E., Hagberg, J.M., Brooke, M.H. and Shumate, J.B., 1979, Bicycle ergometry and gas exchange measurements in neuromuscular diseases. *Archives of Neurology*, **36**, pp. 457–461.

Devries, M.C. and Tarnopolsky, M.A, 2008, Muscle physiology in healthy men and women and those with metabolic myopathies. *Neurology Clinics*, **26**, pp. 115–148, ix.

Elliot, D.L., Buist, N.R., Goldberg, L., Kennaway, N.G., Powell, B.R. and Kuehl, K.S., 1989, Metabolic myopathies: evaluation by graded exercise testing. *Medicine* (Baltimore), **68**, pp. 163–172.

Flaherty, K.R., Weisman, I.M., Zeballos, J. and Martinez, F.J., 2002, The Role of Cardiopulmonary Exercise Testing for Patients with Suspected Metabolic Myopathies and Other Neuromuscular Disorders. *Progress in Respiratory Research,* **32**, pp. 242–253.

Haller, R.G. and Lewis, S.F., 1984, Pathophysiology of exercise performance in muscle disease. *Medicine and Science in Sports and Exercise*, **16**, pp. 456–459.

Lewis, S.F. and Haller, R.G., 1989, Skeletal muscle disorders and associated factors that limit exercise performance. *Exercise and Sports Science Reviews*, **17**, pp. 67–113.

Sockolov, R., Irwin, B., Dressendorfer, R.H. and Bernauer, E.M., 1977, Exercise performance in 6-to-11-year-old boys with Duchenne muscular dystrophy. *Archives of Physical Medicine and Rehabilitation*, **58**, pp. 195–201.

Taivassalo, T. and Haller, R.G., 2004, Implications of exercise training in mtDNA defects--use it or lose it? *Biochimica et Biophysica Acta*, **1659**, pp. 221–231.

Takken, T., Custers, J., Visser, G., Dorland, L., Helders, P. and de Koning, T., 2005, Prolonged exercise testing in two children with a mild Multiple Acyl-CoA-Dehydrogenase deficiency. *Nutrition and Metabolism* (London), **2**, pp. 12.

CHAPTER NUMBER 35

Establishing Maximal Oxygen Uptake in Young People during a Ramp Cycle Test to Exhaustion

A.R. Barker, A.M. Jones, C.A. Williams, and N. Armstrong

University of Exeter, UK

35.1 INTRODUCTION

Maximum oxygen uptake ($\dot{V}O_{2\,max}$) is recognized as the best single measure of aerobic fitness, although the most appropriate methods to assess and interpret $\dot{V}O_{2max}$ in young people remain controversial (Armstrong and Welsman 1994). As only ~ 20-40% of children performing exercise to exhaustion display a plateau in their $\dot{V}O_2$ response to exercise (Armstrong et al., 1995; Rowland, 1993), the term 'peak $\dot{V}O_2$' ($\dot{V}O_{2peak}$) has been adopted. Consequently, paediatric researchers rely on subjective indicators of intense effort (e.g. facial flushing, sweating, unsteady gait, hyperpnoea) supported by secondary 'objective' criteria (e.g. respiratory exchange ratio [RER], blood lactate and heart rate values) to verify a 'maximal' response.

A ramp based cycling protocol is becoming a popular method for determining $\dot{V}O_{2max}$ both in healthy and diseased children (e.g. Barker et al., 2008; Stevens et al., 2009). However, it remains to be established whether the highest $\dot{V}O_2$ attained during ramp cycling exercise reflects a 'true' $\dot{V}O_{2max}$, as determined from supra-maximal exercise testing. Moreover, a recent study has questioned the validity of using secondary criteria during ramp exercise, as RER, heart rate and blood lactate criteria can underestimate $\dot{V}O_{2\,max}$ by 30-40%, or falsely reject a valid $\dot{V}O_{2\,max}$ measure (Poole et al., 2008). As large inter-individual variations in RER (0.95-1.15), heart rate (185-215 beats·min⁻¹) and blood lactate (3-12 mM) are present in children at $\dot{V}O_{2\,max}$ (Armstrong and Welsman 1994), it is plausible that the utility of secondary criteria are equally inappropriate in young people.

The aims of this study were to test the following hypotheses: 1) that using secondary criteria can result in the acceptance of a 'sub-maximal' $\dot{V}O_{2max}$ during ramp cycling exercise in children; and 2) that the highest $\dot{V}O_2$ recorded during a ramp cycling exercise in children is comparable to the highest $\dot{V}O_2$ achieved during supra-maximal testing, thus satisfying the plateau requirement for a 'true' $\dot{V}O_{2max}$.

35.2   METHODS

35.2.1 Experimental design

Thirteen 9-10 y old children (8 boys, 5 girls) completed two tests to exhaustion within a single day on an electronically braked cycle ergometer (Lode, Groningen, Netherlands). The first test consisted of a ramp exercise test to exhaustion to determine their $\dot{V}O_2$ max using a ramp rate of 10 W·min^{-1}. Following a recovery period consisting of 10 min cycling at 10 W and 5 min rest, the participants completed a supra-maximal bout to exhaustion with the intensity set to 105% of the peak power achieved during the ramp test. Oxygen uptake (EX671, Morgan Medical, Kent, UK) was determined every 15 s and a finger tip capillary blood was analysed for lactate concentration following the ramp test (YSI 2300, Yellow Springs, Ohio, USA).

35.2.2 Criteria for establishing maximal oxygen uptake

A plateau in the $\dot{V}O_2$ profile during the ramp test was identified by examining the profile of the residuals against a linear regression extrapolated from the 'linear' portion of the response to end exercise. The secondary criteria used to verify a 'maximal' $\dot{V}O_2$ were an RER of 1.00, a heart rate of 195 beats·min^{-1} and within 85% of age predicted maximum (220-age), and a blood lactate concentration of ≥ 6 mM (Armstrong and Welsman, 1994; Dencker *et al.*, 2007; Leger, 1996; Rowland, 1993).

35.2.3 Statistical analysis

Boys' and girls' data were grouped (n=13) to form a single data set for analysis. Paired samples t-tests examined mean differences between outcome variables with the Bonferroni correction applied for multiple comparisons. Limits of agreement analyses were used to establish the mean bias and 95% confidence limits between the ramp and supra-maximal test responses. The alpha level was set at 0.05.

35.3   RESULTS

Four participants had a $\dot{V}O_2$ plateau at exhaustion, whereas seven showed a linear and two showed an accelerated response. At exhaustion the mean RER was 1.11 [SD 0.06, range 0.99-1.20]. A single boy failed to reach the RER criterion. In the 12 participants that satisfied this criterion, the $\dot{V}O_2$ recorded at an RER of 1.00 (1.293 L·min^{-1} [SD 0.265]) significantly underestimated the $\dot{V}O_2$ recorded at exhaustion (1.681 L·min^{-1} [SD 0.295], P=0.002), representing 77% of the latter.

Mean heart rate at exhaustion was 202 beats·min^{-1} [SD 7, range 191-214]. All children satisfied the 85% of their age predicted maximum criterion (equivalent to ~ 179 beats·min^{-1}). Three children failed to reach the 195 beats·min^{-1} criterion, despite a clear plateau in $\dot{V}O_2$ at exhaustion in 2 of these participants. In the participants that satisfied the heart rate criteria, the $\dot{V}O_2$ recorded at 85% of their age predicted maximum (1.345 L·min^{-1} [SD 0.228]) and at 195 beats·min^{-1} (1.556 L·min^{-1} [0.265]) significantly underestimated the $\dot{V}O_2$ recorded at exhaustion (1.690 L·min^{-1} [SD 0.284] and 1.721 [SD 0.318] respectively; $P<0.002$), representing 80% and 90% of the latter.

Mean blood lactate following ramp exercise was 6.7 mM [SD 2.1, range 4.2-12.1]. Six children (4 boys, 2 girls) satisfied the blood lactate criterion of $\geq$ 6 mM. Of the 7 participants who had a blood lactate < 6 mM, 2 had a plateau in their $\dot{V}O_2$ profile.

Supra-maximal testing yielded a $\dot{V}O_{2\,peak}$ that was not significantly different from the ramp test (1.615 L·min^{-1} [SD 0.307] vs. 1.690 L·min^{-1} [SD 0.284], $P=0.090$, respectively), despite exercising at a higher power output (127 vs. 120 W). The limits of agreement for the $\dot{V}O_{2\,peak}$ achieved during supra-maximal and ramp exercise found a mean bias of -0.075 L·min^{-1}, which corresponds to ~ 4% of the initial ramp test $\dot{V}O_{2\,peak}$ score (95% confidence limits: -0.263 to 0.112 L·min^{-1} or -16 to 6%).

35.4 CONCLUSION

The main findings from the current study are that during ramp cycling exercise in a group of healthy 9-10 year old children: 1) a plateau in the $\dot{V}O_2$ profile at exhaustion is an infrequent phenomenon, occurring in ~ 30% of children; 2) adherence to commonly used secondary criteria to validate a maximal effort in young people can result in either a 'sub-maximal' $\dot{V}O_{2\,max}$ or a rejection of a participant's $\dot{V}O_{2\,max}$ score despite a plateau being evident; and 3) supra-maximal testing at 105% of the power output achieved during ramp exercise did not increase the $\dot{V}O_{2\,peak}$ achieved compared to the ramp test, thus suggesting the achievement of a 'true' $\dot{V}O_{2\,max}$ during the initial ramp test.

Collectively these results provide a basis for paediatric researchers to abandon the use of secondary criteria to validate a 'maximal' $\dot{V}O_2$. Rather, as supra-maximal testing elicits a $\dot{V}O_{2\,peak}$ similar to the ramp protocol, thus satisfying the plateau criterion despite only being present in 30% of the initial ramp responses, it is recommended that the use of such tests should be adopted as *the* appropriate method of confirming a 'true' $\dot{V}O_{2\,max}$ in healthy young people.

35.5 REFERENCES

Armstrong, N. and Welsman, J.R., 1994, Assessment and interpretation of aerobic fitness in children and adolescents. In *Exercise and Sport Science Reviews*, **22**, Holloszy, J.O (Ed). pp. 435–476.

Armstrong, N., Kirby, B.J., McManus, A.M. and Welsman, J.R., 1995, Aerobic fitness of prepubescent children. *Annals of Human Biology*, **22**, pp. 427–441.

Barker, A.R., Welsman, J.R., Fulford, J., Welford, D., Williams, C.A. and Armstrong, N., 2008, Muscle phosphocreatine and pulmonary oxygen uptake kinetics in children at the onset and offset of moderate intensity exercise. *European Journal of Applied Physiology*, **102**, pp. 727–738.

Dencker, M., Thorsson, O., Karlsson, M.K., Linden, C., Eiberg, S., Wollmer, P. and Andersen, L.B., 2007, Gender differences and determinants of aerobic fitness in children aged 8-11 years. *European Journal of Applied Physiology*, **99**, pp. 19–26.

Leger, L. 1996, Aerobic performance. In *Measurement in Pediatric Exercise Science*, edited by Docherty, D., (Human Kinetics, Champaign, Ilinois), pp. 183–224.

Poole, D.C., Wilkerson, D.P. and Jones, A.M., 2008, Validity of criteria for establishing maximal O_2 uptake during ramp exercise tests. *European Journal of Applied Physiology*, **102**, pp. 403–410.

Rowland, T.W., 1993, Does peak $\dot{V}O_2$ reflect $\dot{V}O_2$ max in children?: evidence from supramaximal testing. *Medicine and Science in Sports and Exercise*, **25**, pp. 689–693.

Stevens, D., Oades, P.J., Armstrong, N. and Williams, C.A., 2009, Early oxygen uptake recovery following exercise testing in children with chronic chest diseases. *Pediatric Pulmonology*, **44**, pp. 480–488.

Note

At the time of writing the full version of this paper is *in press* in the *British Journal of Sports Medicine*, but published on-line (doi:10.1136/bjsm.2009.063180), and this extended abstract is reproduced here with permission from the BMJ Publishing Group.

Power Results Normalization in Arm Cranking and Cycloergometer Wingate Tests Performed by Different Matured Swimmers

S. Soares, R.J. Fernandes, J.A. Maia, and J.P. Vilas-Boas

University of Porto, Faculty of Sport, Cifi2d, Portugal

36.1 INTRODUCTION

Performance measures scaling is one fundamental procedure to carry out before making comparisons. For instance, when force or power measures are assessed, weight is often used as a normalization factor. Although, this need for the normalization of the force and power values is not a finished discussion, and the use of the body weight is not unanimously accepted. Indeed, it has not yet been answered if the possible insufficiency of the weight parameter as a normalization factor is independent of performance, especially regarding the test used. Besides weight, other normalization factors like height, limb mass and body mass index (obtained from skin folds, bioimpedance or DEXA) were successfully used (e.g. Mochizuki *et al.*, 2003; Nishio *et al.*, 1992; Raftopoulos *et al.*, 2000).

Wingate test is probably the most widely used method for anaerobic performance evaluation (Van Praagh, 1996) from which are obtained absolute and normalized weight power values. Normalization using body weight is well accepted in these standardized tests. Nowadays, the adequacy of this scaling factor when Wingate Tests are performed seems not to be discussed. The present work intends to reflect about that thematic, starting on the idea that effects obtained after weight normalization were similar for Wingate test performed by the same subjects in arm cranking and cycloergometer.

36.2 METHODS

Ninety swimmers of three maturational states (30 pre-pubertal, 30 pubertal and 30 post-pubertal, being 15 males and 15 females in each group) participated in the present study performing two 30s Wingate tests in consecutive days. One of the tests was performed in an adapted arm cranking and the other was the traditional cycloergometer Wingate Test. An ANOVA test was used to compare maximal (max), mean and minimum (min) power (P) values between the three maturational groups and an independent samples t-test was used to compare the same values between genders. Significance was established at 5%. The total number of differences obtained using absolute values was compared with the total number of differences obtained using relative values. Comparisons were made both for absolute and relative values.

36.3   RESULTS

The number of comparisons established for both arm cranking and cycloergometer Wingate Test, using absolute and weight normalized values, could be observed in Table 36.1.

Table 36.1. Comparison of the total number (n) of differences obtained using absolute and relative power values acquired during an arm cranking and a cycloergometer Wingate Test.

	Arm cranking		Cycloergometer	
	absolute	relative	absolute	relative
Pmax	9	7	9	9
Pmean	8	5	9	8
Pmin	8	3	8	7
Total n	25	15	26	24

It could be observed in Table 36.1 that a large number (10) of differences were lost with the normalization of the power values related to the Wingate Test performed in arm cranking. Results of cycloergometer Wingate Test maintained more stable with the weight normalization. Changes were observed for only two comparisons.

In Figures 36.1 to 36.3 results of the Wingate arm cranking test are expressed case by case. Figure 36.1 shows the weight normalization effect in Pmax obtained through the Wingate arm cranking test. With normalization, no more gender differences for the pre-pubertal group were found. Maturational groups maintained their differences for male swimmers, but differences between pre-pubertal and pubertal female groups disappeared.

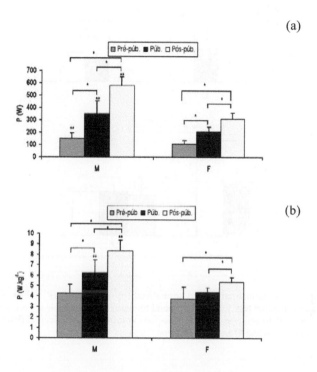

(a)

(b)

Figure 36.1. Non-normalized (a) and normalized (b) maximal power (P) values obtained in a Wingate arm cranking test. Values correspond to male (M) and female (F) pre-pubertal (Pré-púb), pubertal (Púb) and post-pubertal (Pós-púb) swimmers. *significant difference between maturational groups and ** between genders.

Figure 36.2 shows the weight normalization effect in Pmean obtained through the Wingate arm cranking test. Normalization had no effect on gender differences. Although, several maturational group differences disappeared.

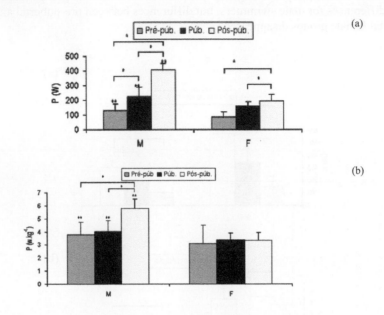

Figure 36.2. Non-normalized (a) and normalized (b) mean power (P) values obtained in a Wingate arm cranking test. Values correspond to male (M) and female (F) pre-pubertal (Pré-púb), pubertal (Púb) and post-pubertal (Pós-púb) swimmers. *significant difference between maturational groups and ** between genders.

Figure 36.3 shows the weight normalization effect in Pmin obtained through the Wingate arm cranking test. Normalization affected both genders and maturational differences. The number of differences lost was higher for maturational groups' comparisons.

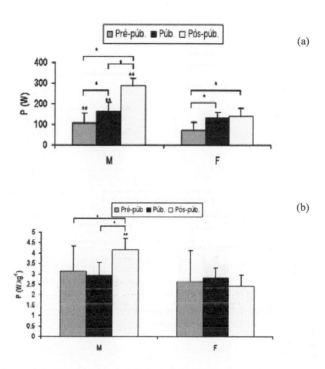

Figure 36.3. Non-normalized (a) and normalized (b) minimum power (P) values obtained in a Wingate arm cranking test. Values correspond to male (M) and female (F) pre-pubertal (Pré-púb), pubertal (Púb) and post-pubertal (Pós-púb) swimmers. *significant difference between maturational groups and ** between genders.

In Figures 36.4 to 36.6 results of the Wingate cycloergometer test are expressed case by case. Figure 36.4 shows that weight normalization had no effect in Pmax values obtained through the Wingate cycloergometer test, both for gender and maturational groups.

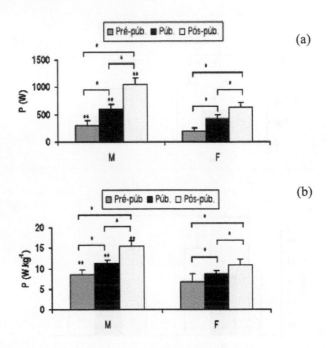

Figure 36.4. Non-normalized (a) and normalized (b) maximal power (P) values obtained in a Wingate cycloergometer test. Values correspond to male (M) and female (F) pre-pubertal (Pré-púb), pubertal (Púb) and post-pubertal (Pós-púb) swimmers. *significant difference between maturational groups and ** between genders.

Figure 36.5 shows that weight normalization had effect in Pmean values obtained through the Wingate cycloergometer test only for female maturational groups. After normalization no more differences between pubertal and post pubertal swimmers were found.

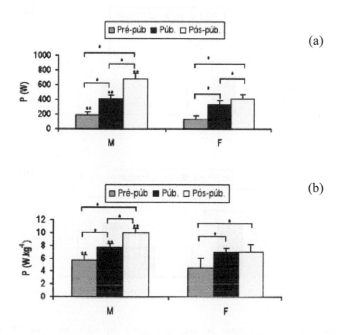

(a)

(b)

Figure 36.5. Non-normalized (a) and normalized (b) mean power (P) values obtained in a Wingate cycloergometer test. Values correspond to male (M) and female (F) pre-pubertal (Pré-púb), pubertal (Púb) and post-pubertal (Pós-púb) swimmers. *significant difference between maturational groups and ** between genders.

Figure 36.6 shows that weight normalization had effect in Pmin values obtained through the Wingate cycloergometer test only for the pubertal group. After normalization gender differences disappeared for this goup.

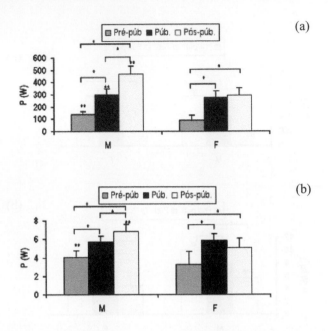

Figure 36.6. Non-normalized (a) and normalized (b) minimum power (P) values obtained in a Wingate cycloergometer test. Values correspond to male (M) and female (F) pre-pubertal (Pré-púb), pubertal (Púb) and post-pubertal (Pós-púb) swimmers. *significant difference between maturational groups and ** between genders.

36.4   CONCLUSION

The aim of this study was to determine the adequacy of the use of body weight as a scaling factor for Wingate tests, performed both in arm cranking and cycloergometer. Weight normalization of the Pmax, Pmean and Pmin values led to results that agree with evidence related to power production by swimmers of different gender and maturational status. Although weight normalization differently affected the three power measures obtained through Wingate test. Weight normalization seemed to affect more Pmean and Pmin, comparatively to Pmax. In fact, this is an interesting result, considering that Pmax is the anaerobic performance indicator generally used in very short duration tests.

When effects of normalization were compared for Wingate performed in arm cranking and cycloergometer, it could be observed that a large number of differences disappeared in Wingate arm cranking comparatively with cycloergometer test performed by the same swimmers. It should therefore be noted that the need for normalization is not equivalent for both tests in which power production is ensured by different body segments. Weight does not seem to be such an accurate normalization factor when power is produced by arms.

Considering maturational groups, it was possible to observe that in Wingate arm cranking, lost differences happened mainly in pre-pubertal swimmers. In Wingate performed in cycloergometer, differences were maintained in this group. This result revealed that for maturational groups' differences the normalization effect was different for different tests.

Thus, the use of body weight as a normalization factor could not always be accurate for inter group comparisons (especially for Pmax). The present study shows that the effects of weight normalization vary with both the test performed (Wingate arms vs cyclo) and swimmers' maturation (more effect on pre-pubertal group). These facts are of particular concern, once studies conclusions are dependent of statistical results.

36.5 REFERENCES

Mochizuki, L., Bianco, R., Brandina, K., Soares, R.J., Oliviera de Cerqueira Soares, S., Albuquerque, J.E., Vargas Avila, A.O., Cerca Serrao, J. and Amadio, A.C., 2003, Efeito da normalização na força de reacção do solo durante a locomoção. *Revista Brasileira de Biomecanica,* **4**, pp. S75–S81.

Nishio, M.L., Madapallimattam, A.G., Jeejeebhoy, K.N., 1992, Comparison of six methods for force normalization in muscles from malnourished rats. *Medicine and Science in Sports and Exercise,* **24**, pp. 259–264

Rattopoulos, D.D., Rabetas, D.A., Armstrong, C.W., Jurs, S.G. and Georgiadis, G.M , 2000, Evaluation of un existing and a new technique for the normalization of ground reaction forces: total body weight versus lean body weight. *Clinical Kinesiology (Online Edition),* **54**, pp. 90–95.

Van Praagh, E.,1996, Testing anaerobic performance. In O. Bar-Or (Ed.), *The child and adolescent athlete*, Blackwell Science, pp. 602–616.

Factors Affecting Leger Shuttle Run Performance in Children

J. Hay[1], and J Cairney[2]

[1]Brock University, Canada; [2]McMaster University, Canada

37.1 INTRODUCTION

Laboratory testing using graded or incremental exercise during which the rate of oxygen uptake is measured continuously is the preferred method of assessing $\dot{V}O_{2max}$ (Armstrong and Welsman, 1997). However, this technique is not feasible for assessing aerobic capacity of large cohorts on repeated occasions. The 20-metre shuttle run test - a progressive, multi-stage, maximal exercise test - was developed to allow a feasible, field-based prediction of peak $\dot{V}O_2$ and has demonstrated moderate to good validity when compared against laboratory assessments (Bono et al., 1991; Boreham et al., 1990; Léger et al., 1988).

Factors that influence test performance are not presently well understood. Although motivation is often cited as a concern influencing test performance (Cairney et al., 2008), anthropometric (e.g., BMI), motoric competence, and behavioural factors (e.g., participation in physical activity) are also likely to influence test performance. Quantification of the relative contribution of the broad range of potential influential factors affecting shuttle run performance is not yet available in the published literature. The aim of this study was to examine the relative contributions of self-efficacy, motivation to performance, anthropometric measures (height, weight, hip and waist girth, leg length), motoric proficiency, physical activity, gender, and age on the Leger shuttle run.

37.2 METHODS

37.2.1 Sample

The study was carried out within the structure of the ongoing PHAST study (Cairney et al., in press) in Ontario, Canada. Children in grade eight from five schools elected at random were assessed in the spring of 2008. A total of 384 children (n=192 males, n=192 females), ages 12 to 14, participated. The Research Ethics Boards of Brock University and the District School Board involved both reviewed and approved the research protocol. Parental consent was obtained for all children.

37.2.2 Testing protocol

Children were first administered two surveys in the homeroom class (CSAPPA, PQ) and then taken from class in smaller groups of 5-10 to complete the shuttle run and anthropometric assessments. Immediately following completion of the Leger test – failure to maintain the required pace – students were directed to a single research assistant to complete a typical 15-point Borg-type rating of perceived exertion (RPE) scale and a similar 15 point rating of perceived motivation (RPM) scale. All assessments were completed by trained research assistants, with the RPM and RPE measures collected by a single trained research assistant.

37.2.3 Shuttle run test

The Léger 20-meter Shuttle Run test (Léger *et al.*, 1984) was used to predict maximal aerobic capacity. The test involves running back and forth between two lines set 20 meters apart in synchrony with a sound signal emitted from an audio compact disc according to previously published procedures. Subjects performed the test in groups of 5-10 subjects and a child's test was complete when unable to maintain the prescribed pace for two consecutive sound signals. We establish aerobic fitness from the last stage completed rather than using the predictive equations as this measure is independent of weight and therefore free from concerns of colinearity. It is closer to an estimation of workload or peak $\dot{V}O_2$.

37.2.4 Psychological, behavioural, anthropometric factors and motor proficiency

The CSAPPA scale is a 20-item scale designed to measure children's generalized self-efficacy toward physical activity (Hay, 1992). A Borg scale for RPE, and a modified Borg scale for RPM were used. Children were shown each scale in turn and indicated their responses by touching it with their finger, doing so out of sight of their peers. The RPM asked children "how hard they had tried to do their best" and response ranged from "didn't try at all" to "tried their very hardest". Physical activity was measured using the Participation Questionnaire (PQ; Hay, 1992).

Height was measured without footwear and with heels together using a SECA™ portable stadiometer. The child was required to stand vertically erect, eyes forward, shoulders relaxed and arms downward. Height was measured and recorded to the nearest 0.2 cm from the highest point on the top of the head. The same procedure was repeated while sitting and sitting height reported allowing leg-length to be determined. Body weight was measured without shoes and wearing light gym clothes and recorded to the nearest 0.1 kg using a Tanita™ electronic scale. Height and mass measurements were used to calculate BMI (kg/m^2) for each participant. Hip and waist girth measures were taken following standard procedures.

Motor proficiency was determined using the results of assessments taken from 2-4 years previously using the Bruininks-Oseretsky Test of Motor Proficiency (BOTMP; Bruininks, 1978). As motor proficiency is a stable construct and very expensive to complete these results were considered acceptable for this analysis.

Age (in years) and gender were collected from self-report.

37.2.5 Statistical analysis

Multiple regressions are used to examine the variance accounted for by *psychological factors* (motivation and exertion, self-efficacy) *anthropometric factors* (hip girth to leg length ratio, BMI), *motor competence* and *physical activity*. Adjusted r-squared values are reported to control for number of variables added to the model. Factors are entered in "blocks" so the unique contribution of each set of variables to overall explained variance can be assessed. Diagnostic tests (variance inflation factors) to ensure multi-collinearity was not a problem were conducted.

37.3   RESULTS

The mean age of the children was 13.4 years (SD=.31). The average BMI for boys was 21.3 (SD=4.18), and for girls, 21.2 (SD=4.18). The average stage completed was 5.4 (SD=2.43) for boys, and 4.0 (SD=1.88) for girls.

In the first part of the analysis, boys and girls are considered together (see Table 37.1). Close to 60% of the total variance is explained by psychological factors, anthropometry, participation in active play, and motor proficiency. Psychological factors (self-efficacy and motivation) account for the greatest proportion of explained variance (43%). Greater hip to leg length ratio and higher BMI were associated with poorer performance. Participation and greater motor proficiency were associated with better test performance.

A parallel analysis was conducted separately for boys and girls. Greater variance in performance was explained by these variables for boys (r^2=.60) than for girls (r^2=.51). BMI (b=-.156; se=.060, p<0.05) and physical activity (b=.129; se=.030, p<0.001) were significant predictors of performance in boys, whereas self-efficacy (b=.054; se=.015, p<0.001) was only significant in girls. Motor proficiency (boys: b=.013; se=.006, p<0.05; girls: =.010; se=.004, p<0.05) and perceived exertion (boys: b=.194; se=.008, p<0.05; girls: =.208; se=.059, p<0.001) were significant predictors of performance for both genders.

Table 37.1. Regression of Leger Stage Completed on Motivation, Self-efficacy, Anthropometry, Participation in Active Play and Motor Proficiency (n=350).

	Model 1	Model 2	Model 3	Model 4	Model 5
Age	.001 (.001)	.001 (.001)	.001 (.001)	.001 * (.001)	.001 (.090)
Girls	-.620 *** (.191)	-1.12 *** (.213)	-1.215 *** (.212)	-.837 ** (.256)	-.256 (.220)
Perceived Exertion	.226 *** (.042)				.232 *** (.048)
Perceived Motivation	.127 *** (.038)				.066 (.039)
CSAPPA	.080 *** (.001)				.039 *** (.011)
Hip-to-leg ratio		-4.60 ** (1.46)			-3.27 * (1.48)
BMI		-.128 ** (.044)			-.104 * (.044)
PQ total			.140 *** (.017)		.072 *** (.021)
Motor Proficiency				.030 ** (.004)	.011 ** (.004)
Adjusted r-squared	.432	.320	.240	.200	.578

*** p<.001, **p<.01, * p<.05; Note: Unstandardized b-coefficients and standard errors (in parentheses) are reported.

37.4   CONCLUSION

The prediction of performance on the shuttle run test was remarkably dependent on psychological and motivational variables, which we have previously demonstrated (Cairney *et al*., 2008). However, it is also evident that anthropometric factors, especially hip to leg ratio, which could influence turning ability, and BMI, which when higher increases the demand of weight on transport, are also significant, although of lesser importance. Interestingly, overall perceived self-efficacy toward physical activity was a predictor of performance for girls but not boys. BMI was only predictive of performance in boys.

37.5 REFERENCES

Armstrong, N. and Welsman, J., 1997, *Young people and physical activity*. Oxford: Oxford University Press.

Bono, M.J., Roby, J.J., Micale, F.G., Sallis, J.F., Shepard, W.E., 1991, Validity and reliability of predicting maximum oxygen uptake via field tests in children and adolescents. *Pediatric Exercise Science*, **3**, pp. 250–255.

Boreham, C.A.G., Paliczka, V.J., Nichols, A.K., 1990, A comparison of the PWC170 and 20-MST tests of aerobic fitness in adolescent school children. *Journal of Sports Medicine and Physical Fitness*, **30**, pp. 19–23.

Bruininks R.H., 1978, *Bruininks-Oseretsky test of motor proficiency owner's manual*. Circle Pines, MN: American Guidance Service.

Cairney, J., Hay, J.A., Faught, B.E., Léger, L. and Mathers, B., 2008, Generalized self-efficacy and performance on the 20-metre shuttle run. *American Journal of Human Biology*, **20**, pp. 132–138.

Cairney, J. and Hay, J.A., Veldhuizenn S., Missiuna, C. and Faught, B.E., Developmental coordination disorder, gender and the activity deficit over time: a longitudinal analysis. *Developmental Medicine and Child Neurology*, in press.

Hay, J.A., 1992, Adequacy in and predilection for physical activity in children. *Clinical Journal of Sports Medicine*, **2**, pp. 92–101.

Léger, L., Mercier, D., Gadoury, G. and Lambert, J., 1988, The multi-stage 20-metre shuttle run test for aerobic fitness. *Journal of Sports Sciences*, **6**, pp. 93–101.

Léger, L., Lambert, J., Goulet, A., Rowna, C. and Dinelle, Y., 1984, Capacité aerobic des Quebecois de 6 a 17 ans Test navette de 20 métres avec paliers de 1 minute. *Canadian Journal of Sports Sciences*, **14**, pp. 21–26.

The Test/re-Test Reliability of Field-Based Fitness Tests in 9-10 Year Old Schoolchildren

L.M. Boddy, G. Stratton, and A.F. Hackett

Liverpool John Moores University, UK

38.1 INTRODUCTION

Accurately assessing the physical fitness of today's children and youth represents an important public health priority, particularly when considering the current obesity 'epidemic', its associated health impacts, and evidence that suggests that poor physical fitness is an independent risk factor for a number of diseases and disorders (Ortega *et al.*, 2008). Ensuring reliability or minimal measurement error during assessments of anthropometrics and fitness is an important consideration for any practitioner who aims to collect meaningful data, particularly when informing policy.

Field-based fitness testing has been used extensively in the past to assess the physical condition of adults and children in large scale studies internationally (Ekblom *et al.*, 2005), with the EUROFIT (Adam *et al.*, 1998) testing battery being widely used in Europe. The Liverpool *Sports*Linx project has used the EUROFIT (Adam *et al.*, 1998) fitness testing battery and an additional test of muscular endurance (speed bounce) from 1998 to the present day to assess skill and health related fitness in three-to-four-thousand 9-10 year old children annually (Taylor *et al.*, 2004). Previous evidence has described acceptable levels of reliability for selected EUROFIT tests (Docherty, 1996). To date, no test/re-test reliability values have been published for the entire test battery used in the *Sports*Linx project and few studies have assessed the individual reliability and limits of agreement for the field-based tests. Therefore the aim of this study was to investigate the test/re-test reliability of the *Sports*Linx field-based fitness testing battery using limits of agreement as well as traditional correlation analyses.

38.2   METHODS

38.2.1 Participants and procedures

Methods used on the *Sports*Linx field based fitness testing have been described elsewhere (Taylor *et al.*, 2004). Briefly, all primary schools in the Liverpool Local Education Authority (LEA) are annually invited to participate in the project. Participants attend a fitness testing session called a 'Fitness Fun Day' where a battery of fitness tests is completed. Experienced Liverpool City Council Fitness Officers lead testing sessions assisted by Liverpool John Moores University Sports Development students. All students involved in the study undergo full training and familiarisation prior to any involvement in testing.

For this study, three schools over two academic years participated in a test re-test analysis. The study has institutional ethical approval. All schools were tested in early November 2006 and 2007. Participants were 9-10 years old (mean age: 9.6 ± 0.3 years) and attended two fitness fun days one week apart. Group, order, venue, day, time, equipment and Fitness testing personnel were standardised between test and re-test. Participants were familiarised with tests and allowed a practice attempt (with the exception of the 20m multi-stage shuttle runs test) prior to recording results. Fitness tests were taken from the EUROFIT (Adam *et al.*, 1998) test battery, with an additional test included to assess muscular endurance (speed bounce) and completed using standard techniques (Taylor *et al.*, 2004). The testing measured aspects of skill and health-related fitness, and the battery consisted of the following measures/tests: stature, body mass, triceps and subscapular skinfold thicknesses, hand grip strength, sit and reach, standing broad jump, 10 × 5m sprints, speed bounce, plate tapping and the 20mMST.

38.2.2 Statistical analysis

Analyses were completed separately for boys and girls. Limits of agreement statistics were employed to assess within-subject test re-test variation. Cronbach's α, and intraclass correlation coefficient (ICC) analyses were completed using SPSS version 14. Correlations were deemed appropriate as the sample was suitably homogenous to avoid the sensitivities associated with correlations and the heterogeneity of participants (Hopkins, 2000), and this analysis provided an indication of relative reliability (Atkinson and Nevill, 1998).Values of ≥0.8 for Cronbach's α and ICC analysis were deemed acceptable levels of reliability for individual and group measures.

38.3   RESULTS

One-hundred and sixty six 9-10 year old participants (91 boys, 75 girls) completed re-test analysis out of 171 (92 boys, 79 girls) original participants (97.1%). Table 38.1 displays mean data and limits of agreement for the fitness measures at test and re-test separated by sex. Cronbach's α and ICC analysis described acceptable levels of reliability for most tests, particularly at the group level, including

20mMST (Table 38.2), however some of these tests exhibited wide LOAs despite acceptable ICC results.

Table 38.1. Mean test and re-test results with limits of agreement for boys and girls.

Measure	Mean Test		Mean Re-test		95% Limits of Agreement	
	Boys	Girls	Boys	Girls	Boys	Girls
Stature (cm)	137.2	138.1	137.5	138.2	-2.7 to 1.9	-2.5 to 2.1
Body mass kg)	34.2	35.7	33.8	36	-4.3 to 4.3	-3.5 to 3.8
BMI (kg/m^2)	17.9	18.5	17.6	18.6	-2.4 to 3.0	-1.2 to 2.7
Triceps Skinfold (mm)	13.5	17.2	13.9	17.6	-2.87 to 2.0	-3.6 to 2.9
Subscapular Skinfold (mm)	9.5	11.6	9.1	11.8	-2.5 to 1.9	-3.5 to 2.5
20mMST (shuttles)	37.5	26.1	40	24	-22.8 to 17.8	- 18.3 to 22.5
Right Hand Grip Strength (kg)	16.2	15.3	15.7	14.5	-4.6 to 5.7	-3.8 to 5.3
Left Hand Grip Strength (kg)	16.7	14.5	15.1	13.8	-4.4 to 5.4	-4.4 to 5.8
Sit and Reach (cm)	15.9	17.9	15.8	17.2	-8.6 to 8.8	-8 to 9.5
10 x 5m Shuttle Runs (seconds)	22.7 s	24.2	22.2	24.7	-4.3 to 3.5	-4.1 to 3.1
Standing Broad Jump (cm)	132	115	126.9	109.7	-28.3 to 38.6	-26.2 to 36.9
Speed Bounce (bounces)	20.3	21.5	23	22.3	-10.9 to 5.5	-7.2 to 5.7
Plate Tapping (seconds)	14.8	14.5	15.1	14.9	-6.8 to 6.1	-6 to 5.2

Table 38.2. Reliability results for fitness measures.

Measure	Cronbach's α		ICC for Average Measures		ICC for Single Measures	
	Boys	Girls	Boys	Girls	Boys	Girls
Stature	0.99	0.99	0.99	0.99	0.98	0.98
Body mass	0.98	0.99	0.98	0.99	0.95	0.99
BMI	0.96	0.99	0.96	0.99	0.91	0.99
Triceps Skinfold	0.99	0.98	0.99	0.98	0.98	0.97
Subscapular Skinfold	0.99	0.99	0.99	0.99	0.99	0.99
20mMST	0.91	0.88	0.91	0.88	0.83	0.78
Right Hand Grip Strength	0.84	0.88	0.84	0.88	0.72	0.78
Left Hand Grip Strength	0.82	0.83	0.82	0.83	0.69	0.71
Sit and Reach	0.73	0.92	0.73	0.92	0.57	0.86
10 x 5m Shuttle Runs	0.72	0.82	0.72	0.82	0.57	0.69
Standing Broad Jump	0.85	0.72	0.85	0.72	0.74	0.56
Speed Bounce	0.78	0.91	0.78	0.91	0.64	0.83
Plate Tapping	0.31	0.49	0.31	0.49	0.18	0.32

38.4   CONCLUSION

The aim of this study was to investigate the test/re-test reliability of the *Sports*Linx field-based fitness testing battery. This study describes acceptable levels of reliability for the majority of the field-based *Sports*Linx fitness tests. These tests are suitable for use when assessing group results and population trends. However results suggest that caution should be urged when assessing individual motor performance on tests that exhibited wide LOAs or low single measure correlations. These findings may have implications for health screening and talent identification programmes that use similar methods to assess children. Such programmes may benefit from including more objective measures of fitness (e.g. $\dot{V}O_{2peak}$). Furthermore, tests that exhibited wide LOAs but acceptable ICC values may warrant further investigations for reliability.

From an epidemiological perspective, where components of fitness represent key determinants of health, the results of this study suggest field-based assessments of fitness are appropriate to assess population trends, and their use is urged to assess the physical condition of children.

38.5   REFERENCES

Adam, C., Klissouras, V., Ravazzolo, M., Renson, R. and Tuxworth, W., 1998, EUROFIT: European test of physical fitness. Rome: Council of Europe, Committee for the Development of Sport.

Atkinson, G. and Nevill, A.M., 1998, Statistical methods for assessing measurement error (reliability) in variables relevant to sports medicine. *Sports Medicine*, **26**, pp. 217–238.

Docherty, D., 1996, *Field Tests and Test Batteries*. Human Kinetics, Champaign, IL.

Ekblom, O., Oddson, K. and Ekblom, B., 2005, Physical performance and body mass index in Swedish children and adolescents. *Scandinavian Journal of Nutrition*, **49**, pp. 172–179.

Hopkins, W.G., 2000, Measures of reliability in sports medicine and science. *Sports Medicine*, **30**, pp. 1–15.

Ortega, F.B., Ruiz, J.R., Castillo, M.J. and Sjostrom, M., 2008, Physical fitness in childhood and adolescence: a powerful marker of health. *International Journal of Obesity*, **32**, pp. 1–11.

Stratton, G., Canoy, D., Boddy, L. M., Taylor, S. R., Hackett, A. F. and Buchan, I.E., 2007, Cardiorespiratory fitness and body mass index of 9-11-year-old English children: a serial cross-sectional study from 1998 to 2004. *International Journal of Obesity*, **31**, pp. 1172–1178.

Taylor, S., Hackett, A., Stratton, G. and Lamb, L., 2004, SportsLinx: Improving the health and fitness of Liverpool's youth. *Education and Health*, **22**, pp. 3–7.

Part VII

Physical Activity

Empirical Evidence to Inform Decisions Regarding Identification of non-Wear Periods from Accelerometer Habitual Physical Activity Data

A.V. Rowlands, D.W. Esliger, J. Eady, and R.G. Eston

School of Sport and Health Sciences, University of Exeter, UK

39.1   INTRODUCTION

Accelerometers are currently the recommended tool for the assessment of physical activity in children (Rowlands, 2007). However, there are recognised limitations to the assessment of activity using accelerometry, one of which is the separation of periods when participants are sedentary from those when the monitor has been removed. When interpreting accelerometer output, it can be difficult to determine whether a string of zeros results from monitor removal or from inactivity. This is an important question because if the person has been sedentary and the data are misclassified as monitor removal, sedentary time will be underestimated and mean activity level may be overestimated. Alternatively, if the person has removed the monitor and engaged in some activity and this is misclassified as sedentary time, then sedentary time will be overestimated and mean activity will be underestimated. With the current increasing public health focus on sedentary time this question is particularly pertinent.

Various criteria have been used to distinguish between monitor removal and sedentary time. For example, Eiberg et al. (2005) and Mattocks et al. (2008) used a period of ten consecutive minutes of zeros to identify that the monitor had been removed in studies of 6-7 y olds and 11-12 y olds, respectively. Anderson et al. (2005) ruled that a period of 20 minutes of consecutive zeros indicated that the monitor had been removed in a study of 13-14 y olds. When analysing the NHANES 2003-04 data, Troiano et al. (2008) used a period of 60 minutes of consecutive zeros to indicate monitor removal in both the children's and the adult's data. Van Coervering et al. (68) stipulated that 180 minutes of continuous zeros indicated monitor removal in 11-14 y olds.

There is clearly variability in the criteria used and there is little empirical evidence as to the most biologically plausible duration of consecutive zeros and whether this differs by age. However, Esliger and colleagues (2005) showed that the 95% CI for the longest motionless bout was 17.5 min in 8-13 y old children who wore the monitor for the entire day. On the basis of this they reported that periods of 20 min or more of consecutive zeros were unlikely if the monitor was worn and could thus be taken to indicate monitor removal. Recently, Evenson and Terry (2009) investigated the impact of different wearing time criteria on activity outcome variables in 182 women postpartum and 204 women 12 months postpartum. Based on the pattern of monitor removal indicated by using criteria of 20 minutes, 40 minutes and 60 minutes of consecutive zeros, they concluded that 60 minutes was the optimum criteria in this population.

An alternative, and complementary, approach to this question is to record the longest period of zeros recorded by accelerometers when people are engaged in a popular seated sedentary activity in a controlled environment. This type of study would inform how long it is biologically plausible for an accelerometer to record zero counts while the monitor is being worn by a person who is seated.

The aim of this study was to determine how many consecutive zeros are recorded by the ActiGraph (the market leader in accelerometry) during a prolonged seated period of time in boys and adults. Results from this study could then be used to inform decisions regarding when to label consecutive zeros as missing data and when to classify it as sedentary time. The selected activities involved watching a film at a cinema or a play at a theatre.

39.2   METHODS

39.2.1 Participants

Twenty-four boys (age: 14.8 ± 0.5 y; height: 1.75 ± 0.09 m; mass: 64.2 ± 10.5 kg) and 23 adults (18 men (age: 24.2 ± 8.8 y; height: 1.76 ± 0.09 m; mass: 74.9 ± 10.0 kg) and 5 women (age: 35.6 ± 15.0 y; height: 1.73 ± 0.12 m; mass: 64.8 ± 11.3 kg)) gave their written informed consent to participate in this study. Parents or guardians of participants under 18 y of age also provided written informed consent. Participants self-reported their height and mass. The procedures were approved by the School Ethics committee and were in accordance with the Helsinki Declaration of 1975, as revised in 1983.

39.2.2 Procedure

Participants wore a uniaxial accelerometer on a belt around the waist and positioned over the right hip. Participants either watched a film at the cinema or a play at the theatre on one of five measurement occasions. Data collection for 20 of the 23 adult participants took place on one of four separate occasions at a cinema in Exeter, U.K. Screenings lasted between 95 and 120 minutes. Data from the remaining three adult participants and all the boys' data were obtained during one school theatre trip in Ipswich, U.K. The theatre show lasted 64 minutes, followed by an 18 minute interval and then a further 44 minute show. No individual left their seat during the show; however the boys sometimes left their seat during the interval period. Participants were instructed to wear the accelerometer for the entire duration of the show and to behave normally.

39.2.3 Physical activity assessment

The ActiGraph unixial accelerometer (GT1M ActiGraph, Monrovia, CA) was programmed to record activity in 1 s epochs. ActiGraph data were processed using Kinesoft software.

39.2.4 Statistical analysis

All data were analysed separately for boys and adults. Descriptive statistics were calculated for all variables. Accelerometer data were analysed to determine the longest period of consecutive zeros and the number of strings of zeros lasting longer than 10, 20, 30 and 60 minutes. These time periods were chosen to represent the criteria frequently used in the literature to distinguish monitor removal from sedentary time. The number of occasions of misclassification of sedentary time as monitor removal was recorded for each of these criteria. Independent t-tests were used to compare the mean maximum duration of consecutive zeros and the number of periods of consecutive zeros lasting more than 10, 20 and 30 minutes recorded by adults to those recorded by the boys.

39.3 RESULTS

Periods of consecutive zeros were significantly longer for adults than for boys (37.7 ± 24.7 cf. 16.0 ± 9.7 minutes, $p < 0.001$). In addition adults accumulated significantly more 10- (3.2 ± 1.7 cf.1.5 ± 1.4, $p < 0.001$), 20- (1.3 ± 1.2 cf. 0.3 ± 0.5, $p < 0.001$) and 30- (0.8 ± 0.9 cf. 0.0 ± 0.2, $p < 0.001$) minute periods of consecutive zeros relative to boys. Use of the 10-minute criterion to classify monitor removal resulted in 74 occurrences of assumed removal in adults (0-6 per adult) and 37 in boys (0-5 per boy). Use of the 20-minute criterion reduced this to 31 occurrences in adults (0-4 per adult) and six in boys (0-2 per boy); the 30-minute criterion reduced this further to 18 occurrences in adults (0-3 per adult) and one in boys. When the 60 minute criterion was used there were 4 misclassifications in adults (0-1 per adult) and no misclassifications in boys.

39.4 CONCLUSION

Several studies in the literature identify strings of consecutive zeros lasting longer than 10 or 20 minutes as monitor removal periods. In this study, these criteria frequently misclassified inactivity as monitor removal. Use of a 30-minute criterion was unlikely to misclassify inactive periods as monitor removal times for boys. The data suggest a longer string of zeros, e.g. 60 minutes as used with the NHANES 2003-04 data (Troiano *et al.*, 2008), and recommended by Evenson and Terry (2009), may be needed to avoid misclassification of inactivity in adults. Further studies should examine the duration of zeros that is biologically plausible during seated time in younger children. As an additional check, when researchers have excluded periods as suspected monitor removal, it is recommended they examine the number of removal periods they have identified in a day in order to examine whether it is likely that the monitor was removed that many times. For example, use of a ten minute period of consecutive zeros to identify monitor removal can lead to an unrealistically high number of removal occasions highlighted in any one day.

39.5   REFERENCES

Anderson, C.B., Hagstromer, M., and Yngve, A., 2005, Validation of the PDPAR as an adolescent diary: Effect of accelerometer cut-points. *Medicine and Science in Sports and Exercise,* **37**, pp. 1224–1230.

Eiberg, S., Hasselstrom, H., Gronfeldt, V., Froberg, K., Svensson, J. and Anderson, L.B., 2005, Maximum oxygen uptake and objectively measured physical activity in Danish children 6-7 years of age: the Copenhagen school child intervention study. *British Journal of Sports Medicine,* **39**, pp. 725–730.

Esliger, D.W., Copeland, J.L., Barnes, J.D. and Tremblay, M.S., 2005, Standardizing and optimizing the use of accelerometer data for free-living physical activity monitoring. *Journal of Physical Activity and Health,* **3**, pp. 366–383.

Evenson, K. and Terry, J.W., 2009, Assessment of differing definitions of accelerometer non-wear time. *Research Quarterly for Exercise and Sport,* **80**, pp. 355–362.

Mattocks, C., Ness, A., Leary, S., Tilling, K., Blair, S.N., Shield, J., Deere, K., Saunders, J., Kirkby, J., Smith, G.D., Wells, J., Wareham, N., Reilly, J. and Riddoch, C., 2008, Use of accelerometers in a large field-based study of children: protocols, design issues, and effects on precision. *Journal of Physical Activity and Health,* **5**, pp. S94–S107.

Rowlands, A.V., 2007, Accelerometer assessment of physical activity in children: an update. *Pediatric Exercise Science,* **19**, pp. 252–266.

Troiano, R.P., Berrigan, D., Dodd, K.W., Mâsse, L.C., Tilert, T. and McDowell, M., 2008, Physical activity in the United States measured by accelerometer. *Medicine and Science in Sports and Exercise,* **40**, pp. 181–188.

Van Coervering, P.L., Harnack, K., Schmitz, J.E., Fulton, D.A. and Galuska, S.G., 2005, Feasibility of using accelerometers to measure physical activity in young adolescents. *Medicine and Science in Sports and Exercise,* **37**, pp. 867–871.

Canada's Report Card on Physical Activity for Children and Youth

R.C. Colley[1,2], M. Brownrigg[2], and M.S. Tremblay[1,2]

[1]Children's Hospital of Eastern Ontario Research Institute, Ottawa, Ontario, Canada; [2]Active Healthy Kids Canada, Toronto, Ontario, Canada

40.1   INTRODUCTION

There is growing evidence and concern that the health of Canadian children has deteriorated in the past few decades and physical inactivity is a powerful contributor. Mass media health promotion campaigns are conducted to influence social norms around health behaviours, including physical activity (PA) (Cavill and Bauman, 2004).

Active Healthy Kids Canada (AHKC; www.activehealthykids.ca) was established in 1994 as a national not for profit organization with a mission *to inspire the nation to engage all children and youth in* PA by providing expertise and direction to policy-makers and the public on how to increase, and effectively allocate resources and attention towards PA for Canadian children and youth. Annually for the past 5 years, the AHKC Report Card (AHKC 2005-2009) has consolidated and translated research knowledge to drive social action for policy change relating to PA among children and youth. To achieve this, the Report Card is in a format that can be easily accessed by media, governments, non-governmental organizations, practitioners and researchers. The Report Card provides a comprehensive assessment of indicators relating to school, family, community and the built environment, and policy that contribute to the PA levels of Canadian children and youth.

40.2   METHODS

40.2.1 Development of indicators

The development of the Report Card began in 2004 when AHKC hosted a symposium with leading issue experts. The purpose of the symposium was to identify key indicators/measures that could be included in the inaugural Report Card. Since 2004, the broad categories of the Report Card have remained consistent however iterations in the indicators within each of these have changed depending on data availability and to reflect the evolving landscape of the issues relating to PA in Canadian children and youth.

40.2.2 Collation of data and information

AHKC works closely with a research work group consisting of experts from across Canada. This work group serves a number of roles including contributing unique data sources, informing the grade assignment process and critically reviewing the Report Card content. The Healthy Active Living and Obesity Research Group (HALO) was established as a research team within the Children's Hospital of Eastern Ontario Research Institute in 2007 and serves as the knowledge partner for the development and writing of the Report Card.

40.2.3 The grade assignment process

The research work group is brought together to evaluate the summation of the evidence each year. Using the framework outlined in Table 40.1, each indicator is evaluated individually and a grade consensus is reached. Key considerations include trends over time, international comparisons, and the presence of disparities (e.g., children with disabilities, geographic differences, socio-economic differences, etc.).

Table 40.1. Grading framework for the Report Card.

Grade	Interpretation
A	We are succeeding with a large majority of Canadian children and youth ($\geq$ 80%).
B	We are succeeding with well over half of Canadian children and youth (60-79%).
C	We are succeeding with about half of Canadian children and youth (40-59%).
D	We are succeeding with less than half but some Canadian children and youth (20-39%).
F	We are succeeding with very few Canadian children and youth (< 20%).

40.2.4 Communications and media strategy

ParticipACTION is a national, not-for-profit, charitable organization incorporated in 1971 with a mission to be the national voice of PA and sport participation in Canada. In 2007, AHKC entered into a strategic communication partnership with ParticipACTION to facilitate dissemination and media outreach of the Report Card across Canada. In essence, ParticipACTION's role is to work with AHKC to optimize knowledge exchange and other evidence-informed communication with the ultimate aim of mobilizing action across government, non-governmental organizations, the media and the public.

40.2.5 Funding structure

Active Healthy Kids Canada has a diverse set of funding partners, relying on multiple funding sources that include contributions from government, and private sector, philanthropic foundation and non-government organization contributions to execute all aspects of its work. In particular, it is striving to grow more effective networks at the provincial-territorial level for in-kind support, further linking to the municipal level through these networks.

40.3 RESULTS

40.3.1 Trends in physical activity

The primary indicator of the Report Card is the state of PA in Canadian children and youth. Since 2007, the AHKC Report Card has reported on objectively measured PA data on Canadian children and youth. These data are collected using pedometers as part of the Canadian Physical Activity Levels Among Youth survey (CAN PLAY) led by the Canadian Fitness and Lifestyle Research Institute (www.cflri.ca).

In 2005-06, 9% of Canadian children and youth were meeting the PA guidelines of 90 minutes of moderate to vigorous PA per day. This value rose to 10% in 2006-07 and again to 13% in 2007-08. The 2009 Report Card suggested cautious optimism was in order given that the rise to 13% could reflect progress but could also reflect aberration in the data from year to year. The annual reporting of these data in the Report Card serves as a critical surveillance instrument and allows AHKC to disseminate the information to a broad range of stakeholders.

40.3.2 Evaluation

In 2008, AHKC commissioned an independent agency to conduct an evaluation of AHKC, its activities and specifically the Report Card considering inputs, activities, outputs, and short, medium and long-term outcomes. Broadly, consideration was given to the Report Card's purpose of raising awareness about the need for PA in children and youth and to motivate decision-makers to enhance opportunities for children and youth to be physically active. The evaluation found that the Report Card is achieving its objective of increasing awareness about PA in children (90% agree) and that the Report Card supports stakeholder mandates (86% agree). Nearly 60% reported using the Report Card for advocacy and policy/strategy development and nearly half reported using it to inform program development, training, and for briefing senior staff and elected officials.

Dissemination and media coverage of the Report Card has grown each year and is facilitated through a provincial/territorial partnership network. In 2009, hard copy distribution surpassed 40,000 copies and media coverage exceeded 100 million media impressions in broadcast (TV and radio), print and online media across Canada.

40.4   CONCLUSION

In May 2008, the Federal-Provincial-Territorial Ministers responsible for Sport, PA and Recreation used data highlighted in the Report Card to set targets to increase the percentage of children and youth meeting PA guidelines and the average number of steps taken daily. In November 2008, their corresponding Deputy Ministers began a process to develop priorities and areas of focus to be coordinated across governments through the Interprovincial-Territorial Sport and Recreation Council PA and Recreation committee, with support from the Public Health Agency of Canada. This led to a joint policy statement aimed an enhancing collaborating to increase PA among children and youth in August 2009. It appears as though the AHKC Report Card has played a key role in informing discussions that have led to action on PA in Canada. Further evidence of the Report Card's influence is in the replication of the model in several other jurisdictions including Saskatchewan, Louisiana, South Africa and Mexico.

40.5   REFERENCES

Active Healthy Kids Canada, 2005, Dropping the ball - Canada's Report Card on Physical Activity for Children and Youth. *Active Healthy Kids Canada*, Toronto, Canada.

Active Healthy Kids Canada, 2006, Canada's Report Card on Physical Activity for Children and Youth. *Active Healthy Kids Canada*, Toronto, Canada.

Active Healthy Kids Canada, 2007, Older but not wiser. Canada's future at risk - Canada's Report Card on Physical Activity for Children and Youth. *Active Healthy Kids Canada*, Toronto, Canada.

Active Healthy Kids Canada, 2008, It's time to unplug our kids – Canada's Report Card on Physical Activity for Children and Youth. *Active Healthy Kids Canada*, Toronto, Canada.

Active Healthy Kids Canada, 2009, Active kids are fit to learn - Canada's Report Card on Physical Activity for Children and Youth. *Active Healthy Kids Canada*, Toronto, Canada.

Cavill, N. and Bauman, A., 2004, Changing the way people think about health-enhancing physical activity: do mass media campaigns have a role? *Journal of Sports Sciences*, **22**, pp. 771–790.

World Health Organization, *The World Health Report, 2002, Reducing Risks, Promoting Healthy Life*, World Health Organization, Geneva.

Dose Related Association of Total Physical Activity and Health-Related Physical Fitness

R. Gruodyte[1,2], V. Volbekiene[2], R. Rutkauskaite[2], and
A. Emeljanovas[2]

[1]University of Tartu, Estonia; [2]Lithuanian Academy of Physical Education, Kaunas, Lithuania

41.1 INTRODUCTION

The beneficial effects of physical activity (PA) to health in adults are well established (Katzmarzyk and Craig, 2006). The influence varies and depends on PA dose and health components. Daily PA is important for children's health, their physical and cognitive development as well as for their physically active behaviour and health in adulthood (Dencker et al., 2006). Low PA in childhood is a risk factor for particular diseases. Physically active children are more physically fit than their physically inactive counterparts. Insufficient physical fitness of adolescents is one of the risk factors for chronic diseases and has a tendency to be carried over into adulthood (Malina, 1996; Renson and Beunen, 2000). Our previous study of 5-11th grade Lithuanian schoolchildren has shown that only 14.2% of boys and girls are meeting the World Health Organisation's guidelines for health-enhancing PA, i.e. 60 min of daily moderate-to-vigorous PA (Volbekiené et al., 2007). We suggest that there is a cause-effect relationship between total volume of PA and health-related physical fitness outcomes in schoolchildren. Nevertheless, further research is needed to identify the most effective dose of PA. The aim of the study was to determine the relationships between total volume of daily PA and health-related physical fitness of adolescent boys.

41.2 METHODS

41.2.1 Experimental design

This cross-sectional study initially recruited 151 healthy, non-obese boys of which 135 have completed all of the required measurements. The participants were all students of a 9th grade (aged 15.2 ± 0.4 years) at randomly selected secondary schools of Lithuania. A full description of the nature of the study has been provided to the boys before obtaining their informed consent. Measurements of PA and health-related physical fitness composed the study protocol.

41.2.2 Physical activity

The total volume of PA was obtained by the modified Short Form of the International Physical Activity Questionnaire (IPAQ) (Ainsworth and Levy, 2004). During the interview, boys were asked to recall the numbers of days per week and time periods (minutes) per day spent in vigorous, moderate, and walking activities. The data of sedentary activities were not included in the study protocol. The total volume of PA, defined as metabolic equivalents (METs) per week, consisted of the amount of energy expended on vigorous, moderate, and walking activities over the last seven days. According to the guidelines (IPAQ, 2005) the boys were divided in three groups: high PA ($\geq$3001 METs/week; n=42), moderate PA (1387-3000 METs/week; n=52); and low PA ($\leq$1386 METs/week; n=41).

41.2.3 Health-related physical fitness

The four components of health-related physical fitness (i.e. cardiorespiratory endurance, muscle strength and endurance, flexibility, and body composition) were measured. Body height was measured on a stadiometer. Body mass, body mass index (BMI), body fat (kg), fat mass %, and lean body mass (kg) were measured using bioelectrical impedance analysis (Tanita BC–418MA). The boys were dressed in light clothing and wearing no shoes.

A battery of physical fitness tests consisted of:
- the Roufier exercise test to assess cardiovascular fitness (Poderys et al., 2005). The participants had to perform 30 squats per 45 s. The heart rate data (pre-, 30s post-, and 2 min post-test) were used to calculate the Roufier index (RI).
- the single maximal vertical jump (cm) to measure the muscle strength of lower limbs (on Kistler forceplate).
- the modified push-up test to determine the muscular endurance of arms and trunk (Suni et al., 1994). The number of correctly performed push ups in 40 seconds was registered.
- the sit-and-reach test to measure flexibility (Eurofit, 1993).

41.2.4 Statistical analysis

Statistical analysis was performed with *MS Excell* and *STATISTICA* programmes. Means and standard deviations were determined. A one-way analysis of variance (ANOVA) and Tukey *post hoc* test were used to compare the differences between the groups. Pearson's product moment correlation was used to examine relationships between total volume of PA and health-related physical fitness components. The level of significance was conducted at $p<0.05$.

41.3   RESULTS

There were no significant differences between the boys in different PA groups in respect of anthropometrical and body composition parameters (Table 41.1).

Table 41.1. Mean (±SD) anthropometrical and body composition parameters of adolescent boys with different physical activity levels.

Group	High PA	Moderate PA	Low PA
N	42	52	41
METs min/week	≥3001	1387-3000	≤1386
Age (yrs)	15.1 ± 0.4	15.2 ± 0.5	15.2 ± 0.4
Height (cm)	179.8 ± 6.0	178.1 ± 6.0	178.3 ± 6.6
Body mass (kg)	66.4 ± 6.3	67.9 ± 11.8	66.2 ± 11.5
BMI (kg/m^2)	20.6 ± 2.1	21.4 ± 3.2	20.7 ± 3.0
Body fat (%)	14.5 ± 3.3	16.3 ± 4.9	15.8 ± 4.2
Fat mass (kg)	9.8 ± 3.0	11.6 ± 5.8	10.8 ± 4.4
Fat free mass (kg)	56.6 ± 4.1	56.4 ± 6.8	55.4 ± 8.1

PA: physical activity; BMI: body mass index

The results of health-related physical fitness in high PA, moderate PA, and low PA groups are presented in Table 41.2. Vertical jump and sit-and-reach tests were performed significantly better by the boys of high PA group. No significant differences were found in Roufier exercise and modified push-up tests between the groups.

Table 41.2. Mean (±SD) anthropometrical and body composition parameters of adolescent boys with different physical activity levels.

	High PA	Moderate PA	Low PA
N	42	52	41
Roufier exercise test (RI)	7.9 ± 4.0	8.1 ± 4.1	8.5 ± 4.5
Vertical jump (cm)	44.2 ± 6.5	40.2 ± 7.3[#]	37.8 + 7.0[#]
Modified push-up (N/40s)	20.1 ± 4.8	18.0 ± 4.9	17.4 ± 4.4
Sit-and-reach (cm)	23.0 ± 6.9	19.6 ± 6.6	16.9 ± 7.1[#]

PA: physical activity; RI: Roufier index; [#]difference from high PA group. $P < 0.05$.

The total volume of PA correlated with muscular strength and endurance, and flexibility in the total group of adolescent boys (r=0.28-0.32, p<0.01). No significant correlations of total volume of PA were found with cardiovascular endurance and body composition (p>0.05).

41.4   CONCLUSION

The results of the present cross-sectional study demonstrated that there is a dose related association between total physical activity and health-related fitness components in healthy adolescent boys. The greater the volumes of total PA, the better are the results of muscle strength of lower limbs and flexibility. Significant correlations of total PA were identified with muscle strength of lower limbs, muscular endurance of arms and trunk, and flexibility in total group of adolescent boys. Although physical fitness in great deal is genetically determined (Bouchard, 1993), it is also dependent on daily PA and health status (Corbin *et al.*, 2000). It is not known at what extent is the influence of daily physical activity on the increase of physical fitness. Although physically active behaviours and health-related fitness are caused by biological heredity, daily PA may have a significant influence on health-related physical fitness of schoolchildren.

41.5 REFERENCES

Ainsworth, B.E. and Levy, S.S., 2004, Assessment of health-enhancing physical activity: methodological issues. In: Oja P, Borms J, editors. *Health enhancing physical activity. Perspectives – the multidisciplinary series of physical education and sport science*, pp. 239–270.

Bouchard, C., 1993, Heredity and health-related fitness. *President's council on physical fitness and sports. Research digest*, **1**, pp. 1–7.

Corbin, C.B., Pangrazi, R.P. and Franks, B.D., 2000, Definitions: health, fitness, and physical activity. *President's council on physical fitness and sports. Research Digest*, **18**, pp. 1–8.

Dencker, M., Thorsson, O., Karlsson, M.K., Lindén, C., Eiberg, S., Wollmer, P. and Andersen, L.B., 2006, Daily physical activity related to body fat in children aged 8-11 years. *Journal of Pediatrics*, **149**, pp. 38–42.

Eurofit. *European tests of physical fitness (2nd edition)*. 1993. Strasbourg.

IPAQ. *The International Physical Activity Questionnaire. Guidelines for data processing and analysis of the International Physical Activity Questionnaire* (IPAQ) – short and long forms. November 2005. Available from: http://www.ipaq.ki.se/.

Katzmarzyk, P.T. and Craig, C.L., 2006, Independent effects of waist circumference and physical activity on risk of all-cause mortality in Canadian women. *Applied Physiology Nutrition and Metab*olism, **31**, pp. 271–276.

Malina, R.M., 1996, Tracing of physical activity and physical fitness across the lifespan. *Research Quarterly for Exercise and Sport*, **67**, pp. 48–57.

Poderys, J., Buliuolis, A., Poderytė, K. and Sadzevičienė, R., 2005, Mobilization of cardiovascular function during the constant-load and all-out exercise tests. *Medicina*, **41**, pp. 1048–1053.

Renson, R. and Beunen, G., 2000, Daily physical activity and physical fitness from adolescence to adulthood: A longitudinal study. *American Journal of Human Biology*, **12**, pp. 487-497.

Suni, J., Oja, P., Laukkanen, R., Miilunpalo, S. and Vartiainen, T.M., 1994, *Test Manual for the Assessment of Health Related Fitness*. Tampere.

Volbekienė, V., Griciūtė, A. and Gaižauskienė, A., 2007, Health-related physical activity of 5-11th grade students from Lithuanian cities. *Education, Physical Training and Sport*, **2**, pp. 71–77.

Comparing Physical Activity Levels of Hungarian Boys and Girls during Weekdays

M. Uvacsek[1], M.Tóth[1], and N.D. Ridgers[2]

[1]Semmelwcis University Budapest, Hungary; [2]Liverpool John Moores University, UK

42.1 INTRODUCTION

In Hungary, the prevalence of overweight and obesity in youth increased from 12% to 28% between 1985 and 2000 (Illyés, 2001). Antal *et al.* (2009) found that prevalence of overweight and obesity were 18.1 and 7.4% for boys and 19.6 and 6.3% for girls, respectively, in 2009. With increasing fatness and obesity in children, the need for increasing physical activity has been highlighted (Uvacsek *et al.*, 2007).

Little objective data have examined the physical activity (PA) levels of Hungarian children using accelerometry, and more data are needed concerning the habitual PA levels of Hungarian children.

This study aimed to examine the physical activity levels of Hungarian children during school days, and to compare the PA levels of boys and girls on each investigated day.

42.2 METHODS

42.2.1 Participants and settings

One hundred fifteen children (mean age = 10.9 ± 1.1; 62% boys; 12% overweight) from 3 public elementary schools in Budapest participated in the study. Each child returned signed informed parental consent. All participating children followed their daily routine. School lessons typically started at 8am and finished between 1-2 pm. In the afternoon, children were able to take part in after school clubs.

42.2.2 Instruments

A hip-mounted uni-axial accelerometer (Actigraph 7164, MTI Health Services, Florida, USA) measured children's physical activity levels every 5 seconds for three consecutive days. The age-specific cut-points that determined time spent in light (LPA), moderate (MPA), and vigorous physical activity (VPA) were derived from the following energy expenditure prediction equation (Freedson et al., 1997):

METS = 2.757 + $(0.0015 \cdot counts \cdot min^{-1})$ – $(0.08957 \cdot age$ [yr]) – $(0.000038 \cdot counts \cdot min^{-1} \cdot age$ [yr])

Moderate-to-vigorous physical activity (MVPA) was calculated by summing MPA and VPA. Time being sedentary was defined as <100 counts per minute (Nilsson et al., 2009). Counts per minute were also obtained for each day. Sustained 20 minute periods of zero counts were deemed to indicate that the accelerometer had been removed. Physical activity data were downloaded using manufacturer software (Actisoft Analysis Software v. 3.2, MTI Health Services) Children who did not achieve min. 600 min wear time/day were excluded from the statistical analysis.

42.2.3 Procedure

Due to equipment availability, 18 children per each week during the investigation had their physical activity quantified across three consecutive days (Wednesday to Friday) between May and October 2008. Participants wore the Actigraph over the right hip using elastic belt. Following a familiarisation session, the children were asked to wear the monitor during all waking hours, except during water-based activities. Prior to attaching the monitors, anthropometric measurements of body mass (to the nearest 0.1kg; Beuer BG22, Beuer, Germany) and stature (to the nearest 0.1cm; Sieber-Hagner, Switzerland) and 7 skinfolds (to the nearest 0.1cm; Lange calliper, USA) were recorded according to the International Biological Program (Weiner and Lourie 1969, Parizkova 1961). BMI and relative body fat content were calculated (Szmodis et al. 1976). Measurements were taken by the same skilled anthropometrist.

42.2.4 Statistical analysis

Standard statistical methods were used for the calculation of means and standard deviations. The gender differences in body dimensions were analysed and the means of each activity level per day were compared across three investigated days, that way we excluded the daily routine difference. Differences between boys and girls were assessed using independent samples t-tests. Statistical analyses were conducted using Statistica for Windows 8.0. Statistical significance was set at p<0.05.

42.3   RESULTS

Descriptive data revealed that boys were significantly older, taller and heavier than girls, though no significant differences were found for body mass index (BMI) and body fat content. Altogether 12% of our children were classified overweight or obese according to Cole *et al.* (2000) classification.

Table 42.1 shows the comparison of physical activity levels of girls and boys across each of the three days. There were significant differences between boys and girls in sedentary time on days 2 and 3, with girls engaging in more sedentary activity than boys. No significant differences in time spent in light activity were observed. Boys engaged in significantly more MPA on day 3, VPA on day 2, and MVPA on days 2 and 3 compared to girls. In addition, boys' CPM were significantly higher on days 2 and 3 than girls'.

Table 42.1. Time spent in different physical activity levels (mean ± SD) of Hungarian girls and boys.

		Girls	Boys	#girls	#boys	p
Sedentary	1.day	490.7±70.4	477.5±109.2	40	69	0.49
	2.day	585.1±76.8	540.3±87.2	41	66	0.00
	3.day	574.5±104.7	508.9±101.0	35	52	0.00
LPA	1.day	174.3±31.0	179.0±44.8	40	69	0.55
	2.day	185.6±31.5	195.5±37.7	41	66	0.16
	3.day	183.0±41.9	197.4±43.4	35	52	0.12
MPA	1.day	87.1±22.4	91.7±29.1	40	69	0.39
	2.day	90.9±29.8	101.2±29.6	41	66	0.08
	3.day	92.3±23.3	106.4±25.8	35	52	0.01
VPA	1.day	44.8±15.3	45.7±26.4	40	69	0.84
	2.day	41.8±22.0	52.0±25.6	41	66	0.03
	3.day	47.3±24.5	53.8±25.3	35	52	0.24
MVPA	1.day	132.0±33.5	137.4±51.2	40	69	0.54
	2.day	132.7±47.6	153.2±50.0	41	66	0.03
	3.day	139.7±43.9	160.3±45.6	35	52	0.03
CPM	1.day	730.6±190.9	852.4±391.2	40	69	0.06
	2.day	657.6±261.5	869.6±342.6	41	66	0.00
	3.day	742.7±290.4	937.3±348.9	35	52	0.00

Note: MVPA is the sum of moderate PA and vigorous PA. Numbers included in analyses across days differ due to children's data being excluded.

42.4   CONCLUSION

Little objective data exist on Hungarian school children's physical activity. Ridgers *et al.* (in press) highlighted that boys were more active during daily recess than girls. These data somewhat support these findings. Some differences were observed in habitual physical activity levels between boys and girls across days. Girls spend more time being sedentary than boys. Boys were more active than girls when MVPA and CPM were considered, particularly during days 2 and 3 (Thursday and Friday). Hungarian children's MVPA was over double the international 60min./day recommendation. The relatively high average of MVPA during weekdays may be explained by the intensive physical education lessons and participation in afternoon clubs in schools, which typically last 90 minutes per day. This study should be repeated in different schools to determine if Hungarian children's PA is higher compared to other countries, and to examine how generalisable these findings are to the rest of the school population in Hungary.

42.5 REFERENCES

Antal, M., Péter, S., Biró, L., Nagy, K., Regoly-Mérei, A., Arató, G., Szabó, C. and Martos, E., 2009, Prevalence of underweight, overweight and obesity on the basis of body mass index and body fat percentage in Hungarian schoolchildren: Representative survey in metropolitan elementary schools. *Annals of Nutrition and Metabolism,* **54**, pp. 171–176.

Cole, T.J., Bellizzi, M.C., Flegal, K.M. and Dietz, W.H., 2000, Establishing a standard definition for child overweight and obesity worldwide: international survey. *British Medical Journal*, **320**, pp. 1–6.

Freedson, P.S., Sirard, J., Debold, E., Pate, R., Dowda, M., Trost, S. and Sallis, J., 1997, Calibration of the Computer and Science Applications, Inc (CSA) accelerometer. *Medicine and Science in Sports and Exercise,* **29**, pp. S45.

Illyés, I., 2001, *Az elhízás mai szemlélete*. (The Modern Approach to Obesity). Medicina, Budapest, Hungary. (Hungarian)

Nilsson, A., Anderssen, S.A., Andersen, L.B., Froberg, K., Riddoch, C., Sardinha, L.B. and Ekelund, U., 2009, Between- and within-day variability in physical activity and inactivity in 9- and 15-year old European children. *Scandinavian Journal of Medicine and Science in Sports,* **19**, pp. 10–18.

Parízková, J. (1961): Total body fat and skinfold thickness in children. *Metabolism,* **10:** 794–807.

Ridgers, N.D., Tóth, M. and Uvacsek, M. Physical activity levels of Hungarian children during recess. *Preventive Medicine* ((in press).

Szmodis, I., Mészáros, J. and Szabó, T., 1976, Alkati és működési mutatók kapcsolata gyermek., serdülő- és ifjúkorban. (The body shape and performance in children, adolescents and in youth) *Testnevelés- és Sportegészségügyi Szemle*, **17**, pp. 255–272. (Hungarian).

Uvacsek, M., Mészáros, J., Mészáros, Z., Kalabiska, I., Sziva, Á. and Vajda, I., 2007, Generation differences in BMI and cardio-respiratory endurance in boys. *Humanbiologia Budapestinensis,* **31**, pp. 139–146.

Weiner, J.E.S. and Lourie, J.A., 1969, *Human Biology. A Guide to Field Methods*. IBP Handbook, No. 9. Blackwell Scientific Publishers, Oxford.

Relations Between Maturity Status, Physical Activity, and Physical Self-Perceptions in Primary School Children

S.J. Fairclough[1,2], and N.D. Ridgers[1,3]

[1]REACH Group, UK; [2]Faculty of Education, Community & Leisure; [3]Research Institute for Sport and Exercise Sciences, Liverpool John Moores University, UK

43.1 INTRODUCTION

Currently, there is a paucity of literature reporting the interplay between physical activity, maturity status, and physical self-perceptions in primary school children. Where such studies exist self-report measures of physical activity and maturity status are often used, but these methods may lack accuracy due to difficulties in interpretation and the risk of socially desirable responses (Welk *et al.*, 2000). The purpose of this study was to assess the influence of maturity status on the physical activity and physical self-perceptions of English primary school children using objective methods.

43.2 METHODS

43.2.1 Participants and instruments

Data were gathered from 10 to 11 year old children from a large town in north-west England. Completed parental consent and child assent were returned from 230 children (116 girls; 74.4% response rate). Ethical approval was obtained from the University Ethics Committee.

Chronological age was calculated by subtracting each child's date of birth from the measurement date. Stature and sitting height were measured to the nearest 0.1 cm using a portable stadiometer. Leg length was calculated by subtracting sitting height from stature. Body mass was measured to the nearest 0.1 kg using calibrated scales.

Somatic maturity status was estimated by determining years from attainment of peak height velocity, which is a common technique used in longitudinal studies (Malina *et al.*, 2004). Years from attainment of peak height velocity for each child were predicted using gender-specific regression equations that included stature, sitting height, leg length, chronological age and their interactions (Mirwald *et al.*, 2002). Years from attainment of peak height velocity were subtracted from chronological age to predict age at peak height velocity.

Physical self-perceptions were assessed using the Children and Youth version of the Physical Self-Perception Profile (Whitehead, 1995). The Children and Youth Physical Self-Perception Profile follows a hierarchical structure with global self-esteem at the apex and physical self-worth positioned at the domain level. Subordinate to physical self-worth are four sub-domains of sport competence (Sport), physical condition (Condition), body attractiveness (Attractiveness), and physical strength (Strength).

Physical activity was objectively measured every 5 seconds for five consecutive days (Friday through to Tuesday) using ActiGraph accelerometers. Data from children with at least 3 valid measurement days (including a minimum of 1 weekend day) were retained for further analysis. The number of minutes of moderate-to-vigorous physical activity were calculated using a moderate intensity cut-point of 2000 counts • min^{-1} (Ekelund *et al.*, 2004).

43.2.2 Data analysis

Descriptive statistics ($M \pm SD$) were initially calculated for all measured variables. A multi-level association model was used to assess the effects of gender on physical activity and physical self-perceptions, after being corrected for age at peak height velocity, socio-economic status, and number on roll. Two analyses were conducted for each outcome variable. The first analysis determined the difference between boys and girls on the outcome variable ('crude' analysis), while the second analysis investigated this difference when the covariates were added to the model ('adjusted' analysis) (Twisk, 2006).

43.3   RESULTS

Boys were slightly taller and heavier than the girls and were also 0.1 years older which though statistically significant (t (173) = 2.5, p = .013), produced only a small effect size (d = 0.33). Girls' predicted age at peak height velocity was 1.6 years earlier than boys' (t (173) = 24.22, p < .0001, d = 3.56). Moderate-to-vigorous physical activity was 19.7% greater in boys compared to girls (Table 43.1). Sixty three percent of boys achieved the recommended 60 minutes of moderate-to-vigorous physical activity per day compared to 30% of girls. The summary statistics for the children's physical self-perceptions are also shown in Table 43.1.

Table 43.1. Descriptive summary of physical activity and physical self-perceptions (M ± SD).

Variable	Boys ($n = 78$)	Girls ($n = 97$)
Physical activity		
MVPA (min)	67.3 (19.5)	54.0 (13.7)
Physical self-perceptions		
Sport	3.13 (0.61)	2.87 (0.58)
Condition	3.14 (0.64)	2.92 (0.60)
Attractiveness	2.80 (0.66)	2.58 (0.67)
Strength	2.96 (0.62)	2.59 (0.56)
PSW	3.08 (0.62)	2.90 (0.65)

In the 'crude' multi-level analyses, gender was a significant positive predictor variable for moderate-to-vigorous physical activity, with boys engaging in 13.52 minutes more activity than girls. When the analyses were adjusted to correct for maturity status the gender difference in moderate-to-vigorous physical activity was reduced to 1.73 minutes and the degree of statistical significance also diminished. Gender was a significant positive predictor for each physical self-perception sub-domain, with physical self-worth also approaching significance ($p = .06$). In each case boys had higher physical self-perceptions than girls with the greatest differences evident for Strength (CI – 0.19 to 0.55) and Sport (CI = 0.09 to 0.43). The adjusted analyses revealed that for Sport, Condition, Attractiveness, and physical self-worth the significant effect of gender was no longer apparent when age at peak height velocity was added to the model. The exception to this trend was Strength, where the extent of the gender differences increased by 36% when maturity status was co-varied into the analysis (CI – 0.21 to 0.95).

Significant interaction terms were found between gender and perceptions of Sport, Condition, and Strength. The pattern of association was that as girls' maturity status advanced their physical-self perceptions decreased, whilst boys' physical-self perceptions increased in line with increasing age at peak height velocity.

43.4   CONCLUSION

Hypothesised gender differences in physical activity and physical self-perceptions were initially observed. However, when the effects of maturity status were controlled, the consequences of the puberty-related changes which influence gender differences in moderate-to-vigorous physical activity and physical self-perceptions were reduced. Furthermore, considering previously reported associations between physical activity and the Children and Youth Physical Self-Perception Profile sub-domains it is possible that the interactions observed in our analysis between gender and maturity status suggest that physical self-perceptions mediated the effects of maturity status on moderate-to-vigorous physical activity. Thus, the combination of biological and psychosocial changes that exert an influence on girls' physical self-perceptions during maturation may lead to a decrease in physical activity, while in boys these changes may result in relatively more positive self-perceptions which are manifested as higher levels of moderate-to-vigorous physical activity. However, further exploration of data from a wider age range is necessary to confirm these suppositions.

43.5   REFERENCES

Ekelund, U., Sardinha, L.B., Anderssen, S.A., Harro, M., Franks, P.W., Brage, S., Cooper, A.R., Andersen, L.B., Riddoch, C. and Froberg, K., 2004, Associations between objectively assessed physical activity and indicators of body fatness in 9 to 10 year old European children: A population-based study from 4 distinct regions in Europe (The European Youth Heart Study). *American Journal of Clinical Nutrition*, **80**, pp. 584–590.

Malina, R. M., Bouchard, C. and Bar-Or, O., 2004, *Growth, Maturation and Physical Activity*. Champaign, IL: Human Kinetics.

Mirwald, R. L., Baxter-Jones, A. D. G., Bailey, D. A. and Beunen, G. P., 2002, An assessment of maturity from anthropometric measurements. *Medicine and Science in Sports and Exercise*, **34**, pp. 689–694.

Twisk, J. W. R., 2006, *Applied Multilevel Analysis*. Cambridge: Cambridge University Press.

Welk, G.J., Corbin, C.B. and Dale, D., 2000, Measurement issues in the assessment of physical activity in children. *Research Quarterly for Exercise and Sport*, **71**, pp. S59-S73.

Whitehead, J. R., 1995, A study of children's physical self-perceptions using an adapted physical self-perception profile questionnaire. *Pediatric Exercise Science*, **7**, pp. 132–151.

Introducing the Canadian Assessment of Physical Literacy

M. Lloyd, and M.S. Tremblay

Children's Hospital of Eastern Ontario Research Institute, The Health Active Living and Obesity Research Group, Canada

44.1 INTRODUCTION

Physical activity is a key determinant of health, and an active lifestyle can positively influence multiple developmental and health domains (Physical Activity Guidelines Advisory Committee, 2008). How can children be expected to lead a healthy active lifestyle if they are not taught the value of a physically active lifestyle, or do not have the skills or understanding of what it means to be fit and active (Delaney et al., 2008; Tremblay and Willms, 2003)? Many children today lack the basic skills, knowledge and physical activity behaviours needed to lead healthy active lifestyles (Delaney et al., 2008) and the evidence is illustrated in the startling obesity rates (Tremblay and Willms, 2003).

The aim of this project is to develop a comprehensive tool to measure physical literacy in Canadian schools thus allowing education, sport, recreation, and health experts to better understand the quality and effectiveness of current programming. The Canadian Assessment of Physical Literacy (CAPL) is being developed to objectively measure the status of physical activity, fitness, motor skill proficiency, and related psychosocial mediators and moderators (e.g. knowledge, attitudes, and preferences) of Canadian school-children. Initially the CAPL is being designed for children in grades 4-6; subsequent versions will assess other grade and age levels.

Physical literacy is conceived to be the foundation skills or tools, social/cognitive, behavioural, and fitness related, that children need to possess or develop in order to receive the inherent health benefits of taking part in physical activity for life-long enjoyment and success (Lloyd et al., in press). Physical literacy is deemed to have four core domains, a) physical fitness (cardio-respiratory, muscular strength and flexibility), b) motor behaviour (fundamental motor skill proficiency), c) physical activity behaviours (objectively measured daily activity), and d) psycho-social/cognitive factors (attitudes, knowledge, feelings) (Lloyd et al., in press). Being physically literate is conceived to be the result of the multi-dimensional interaction of these domains to facilitate lifelong healthy active living behaviours in children and youth. Aggregating these 4

domains together to create a comprehensive assessment of physical literacy has not
been done and is the focus of this work (Figure 44.1).

Figure 44.1. The four domains of the Canadian Assessment of Physical Literacy.

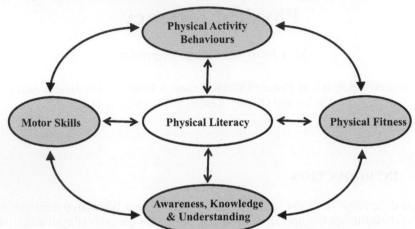

Traditionally, each of the core domains of physical literacy are studied
independently (e.g. fitness separate from movement skills) and are often not
evaluated in any rigorous fashion. Recent research has started to evaluate the
relationship between fitness and motor proficiency and the evidence indicates that
children with more proficient fundamental movement skills engage in more
physical activity and less sedentary behaviour (Fisher *et al.*, 2005; Williams *et al.*,
2008; Wrotniak *et al.*, 2006). Fitness levels also correlate with higher physical
activity levels (Ruiz *et al.*, 2006). Closely linked to the lack of available measures
of physical literacy, is the fact that there is no information on the expected
standards, or measures of competence and this is desperately needed.

44.2   CONCEPTUAL FRAMEWORK

Assessment tools with sound conceptual frameworks demonstrate high construct
validity (Burton and Miller, 1998). For the development of the CAPL we are using
The International Classification of Functioning, Disability and Health model (ICF)
which is the World Health Organization's assessment framework for health and
functioning (WHO, 2001). This model is a valuable tool in research and
assessment because it encompasses multiple domains; it considers functional status
or health status to be the result of the interaction of the *body and its structures,
activity abilities, and participation level* mediated by *personal* and *environmental
factors* (WHO, 2001). Generally, the ICF provides a framework or structure for
assessment research. We believe this is the most appropriate model from which to
frame our work for two reasons, 1) it is a model of health assessment, and 2) it is a
multi-dimensional model that accommodates the reciprocal relationships between

body structures and functions, activity and participation, whiling considering personal and environmental factors, all of which are consistent with the concept of physical literacy. The final version of the CAPL will strive to be *inclusive, adaptable, individualized, safe, complementary, comprehensive and provider friendly.*

44.3 CAPL TEST ITEMS

44.3.1 Motor skills

The motor skills module assesses study participants' performance in both static and dynamic motor skills that are explicitly identified in the Ontario physical education curriculum for grades 4 through 6. Participants demonstrate their proficiency with the following motor skills: throwing, catching, striking (t-ball), kicking (soccer), dribbling, one-leg static balance, and running. Additionally, participants perform jumping, dodging, kicking, hopping, catching, and throwing skills while running through an obstacle course that is timed to allow for a more dynamic and open assessment of fundamental motor skills.

44.3.2 Physical activity behaviour

The CAPL uses pedometers to objectively measure physical activity behaviour. Participants are asked to wear the pedometer on their right hip for seven consecutive days and complete a daily log sheet identifying when the pedometer was put on in the morning, when it was taken off at night, as well as if and why it was removed at any point during the day.

44.3.3 Physical fitness

The fitness module assesses study participants' performance on seven physical and health-related fitness tests. Test items measure cardio-respiratory fitness, muscular strength and endurance, and flexibility. The tasks include: partial curl-ups, push-ups, grip strength, sit and reach, trunk lift, arm flexibility, and the PACER test.

44.3.4 Awareness, knowledge and understanding

The knowledge, awareness and understanding module of the CAPL is the area that requires the most pilot work. Therefore, several iterations of the questionnaire are planned. Question types include fill in the blank, multiple choice, and free response. Answers generated from pilot testing provided much insight into the student's views and opinions about physical activity and health and a second version of the questionnaire is now being tested.

44.4   CONCLUSION

Cycle 1 of pilot testing indicates that it is feasible to create and implement a new assessment of physical literacy. The significant financial support generated quickly from multiple sources (government, health sector, education sector, not-for-profit organizations, and peer-reviewed granting agencies) demonstrates wide-spread interest in this type of data. The success of the pilot testing also indicates substantial support for the CAPL at the grass roots level, among teachers and recreation leaders. Pilot testing will continue and detailed psychometric properties of this new assessment tool will be created to promote widespread use by both researchers and practitioners. Ultimately it is hoped that the CAPL will elevate the importance of careful measuring and monitoring of programs designed to improve physical literacy (e.g. physical education classes, sport lessons, recreation programs) and assist in assessing the efficacy of future interventions.

44.5   REFERENCES

Burton, A.W. and Miller, D.E., 1998, *Movement Skill Assessment*. Champaign, IL: Human Kinetics.

Delaney, B.J., Donnelly, P., News, J. and Haughey, T.J., 2008, *Improving Physical Literacy*. Belfast: Sport Northern Ireland.

Fisher, A., Reilly, J.J., Kelly, L.A., Montgomery, C., Williamson, A., Paton, J.Y. and Grant , S., 2005, Fundamental movement skills and habitual physical activity in young children. *Medicine and Science in Sports and Exercise*, **37**, pp. 684–688.

Lloyd, M., Colley, R. and Tremblay, M., Advancing the Debate on 'Fitness Testing' for Children: Perhaps We're Riding the Wrong Animal. *Pediatric Exercise Science* (in press).

Physical Activity Guidelines Advisory Committee, 2008, Physical Activity Guidelines Advisory Committee Report. Washington, DC: U.S. Department of Health and Human Services.

Ruiz, J.R., Rizzo, N.S., Hurtig-Wennlof, A., Ortega, F.B., Warnberg, J. and Sjostrom, M., 2006, Relations of total physical activity and intensity to fitness and fatness in children: the European Youth Heart Study. *American Journal of Clinical Nutrition*, **84**, pp. 299–303.

Tremblay, M.S. and Willms, J.D., 2003, Is the Canadian childhood obesity epidemic related to physical inacivity? *International Journal of Obesity*, **27**, pp. 1100–1105.

van der Horst, K., Chin A., Paw, M.J., Twisk, J.W.R. and Van Mechelen, W., 2007, A brief review on correlates of physical activity and sedentariness in youth. *Medicine and Science in Sports and Exercise*, **39**, pp. 1241–1250.

WHO, 2001, International classification of functioning, disability and health: ICF. Geneva: World Health Organization.

Williams, H.G., Pfeiffer, K.A., O'Neill, J.R., Dowda, M., McIver, K.L., Brown, W.H. and Pate, R.R., 2008, Motor skill performance and physical activity in preschool children. *Obesity (Silver Spring)*, **16**, pp. 1421–1426.

Wrotniak, B.H., Epstein, L.H., Dorn, J.M., Jones, K.E. and Kondilis, V.A., 2006, The relationship between motor proficiency and physical activity in children. *Pediatrics*, **118**, pp. e1758–1765.

Correspondence Addresses

J.S. Baker
Exercise and Health Sciences
School of Science
University of the West of Scotland
Hamilton Campus, Almada Street
Hamilton ML3 0JB
United Kingdom
E-mail: Julien.baker@uws.ac.uk

G. Baquet
Faculty of Sports Sciences and
Physical Education
9, rue de l'université
59790 Ronchin
France
E-mail: georges.baquet@univ-lille2.fr

A.R. Barker
Children's Health and Exercise
Research Centre
School of Sport and Health Sciences
University of Exeter
Exeter
EX1 2LU
United Kingdom
E-mail: A.R.Barker@exeter.ac.uk

R. Beneke
Department of Biological Sciences
University of Essex
Wivenhoe Park, Colchester
CO4 3SQ
England
United Kingdom
E-mail: rbeneke@essex.ac.uk

S. Berthoin
Faculty of Sports Sciences
9, rue de l'université
59790 Ronchin
France
E-mail: serge.berthoin@univ-lille2.fr

L.M. Boddy
IM Marsh Campus
Liverpool John Moores University
Barkhill Road
Liverpool
L17 6BD
United Kingdom
E-mail: L.M.Boddy@ljmu.ac.uk

B. Borel
EA 3608
Faculté des Sciences du Sport
Université de Lille 2 Droit – Santé
9 rue de l'université
59790 Ronchin
France
E-mail: benoit.borel-2@univ-lille2.fr

B.C. Breese
Children's Health and Exercise
Research Centre
School of Sport and Health Science
University of Exeter
Exeter, United Kingdom
EX1 2LU
E-mail: Bb229@exeter.ac.uk

M.J. Coelho e Silva
University of Coimbra
Faculdade de Ciencias do Desporto e
Educacao Fisica
Estadio Universitario, Pav_III
3040-156 Coimbra
Portugal
E-mail: mjcesilva@fcdef.uc.pt

R.C. Colley
Room 3111, Research Building 2
Healthy Active Living and Obesity
Research Group
Children's Hospital of Eastern
Ontario Research Institute
401 Smyth Road
Ottawa, Ontario, Canada
Canada
K1H 8L1
E-mail: rcolley@cheo.on.ca

J.F. De Groot
Department of Pediatric
Physiotherapy and Exercise
Physiology
Wilhelmina Children's Hospital,
University Medical Center Utrecht
Room kb.02.056.0. P.O. Box 85090,
3508 AB Utrecht
The Netherlands
E-mail: J.F.degroot-
16@umcutrecht.nl

D.R. Dengel
University of Minnesota
111 Cooke Hall
1900 University Avenue S.E.
Minneapolis, MN 55455
USA
E-mail: denge001@umn.edu

A. Eliakim
Child Health and Sports Center
Chair, Pediatric Department
Meir General Hospital
Kfar-Saba, Israel 44821
E-mail: eliakim.alon@clalit.org.il

S.J. Fairclough
Faculty of Education
Community and Leisure
Liverpool John Moores University
United Kingdom
E-mail: s.j.fairclough@ljmu.ac.uk

B. Falk
Faculty of Applied Health Sciences
Brock University
St Catharines
Ontario
Canada
E-mail : bfalk@brocku.ca

D.J. Green
John Moore University, Liverpool
and
School of Sport Science-Exercise
and Health
University of Western Australia,
Australia
E-mail: D.J.Green@ljmu.ac.uk

R. Gruodytė
Faculty of Exercise and Sport
Sciences
Institute of Sport Pedagogy and
Coaching Sciences
Jakobi 5
Tartu 51014
Estonia
E-mail: r.gruodyte@lkka.lt

J. Hay
Professor, Community Health
Sciences
Brock University
500 Glenridge Ave.
St. Catharines, ON Canada
L2S 3A1
E-mail: jhay@brocku.ca

T. Jürimäe
University of Tartu
Faculty of Exercise and Sports
Sciences
Jakobi 5
51014 Tartu
Estonia
E-mail: toivo.jurimae@ut.ee

H.C.G. Kemper
Han CG Kemper, Prof Emeritus
EMGO Institute
VU University Medical Center
van der Boechorststraat 7
1081 BT Amsterdam
The Netherlands
E-mail: hcg.kemper@vumc.nl

E. Leclair
Faculté des Sciences du Sport et de
l'Education Physique (EA3608)
Univ Lille Nord de France
9, rue de l'Université
59790 Ronchin
France
E-mail: leclair.erwan@gmail.com

A.D. Mahon
Human Performance Laboratory
Ball State University
Muncie, IN 47306
USA
E-mail: tmahon@bsu.edu

J.A. Maia
Faculdade de Desporto
University of Porto
Rua Dr. Plácido Costa, 91
4200-450 Porto
Portugal
E-mail: jmaia@fade.up.pt

S. Matecki
INSERM ERI 25
Université de Montpellier 1
Montpellier
France
E-mail: s-matecki@chu-
montpellier.fr

Y. Meckel
Zinman College of Physical
Education and Sport Sciences
Wingate Institute
Netanya, Israel
E-mail: meckel@wincol.ac.il

D. Nemet
Child Health & Sports Center
Department of Pediatrics
Meir General Hospital
59 Tchernichovski St
Kfar-Saba, Israel, 44281
E-mail: dnemet@gmail.com

J. Obeid
Children's Exercise & Nutrition
Centre
Chedoke Hospital, Evel Building,
Room 463A
555 Sanatorium Road
Hamilton, ON, Canada
L8N 3Z5
E-mail: obeidj@mcmaster.ca

R. Pilz-Burstein
Wingate Institute
Netania
Israel
E-mail: rutiepb@wingate.org.il

A.V. Rowlands
Senior Lecturer
School of Sport and Health Sciences
University of Exeter
St. Luke's Campus
Heavitree Road
Exeter EX1 2LU
England, United Kingdom
E-mail: a.v.rowlands@exeter.ac.uk

S. Soares
Rua Dr. Plácido Costa, 91
4200.450 Porto
Portugal
E-mail: susana@fade.up.pt

T. Takken
Department of Pediatric Physical
Therapy & Exercise Physiology
Wilhelmina Children's Hospital
University Medical Center Utrecht
Room KB.02.056.
P.O. Box 85090
NL-3508 AB Utrecht
the Netherlands
E-mail: t.takken@umcutrecht.nl

N.E. Thomas
Centre for Child Research
School of Human Sciences
Swansea University
Singleton Park
Swansea
Wales SA2 8PP
E-mail: n.e.thomas@swansea.ac.uk

K. Tolfrey
School of Sport, Exercise and Health
Sciences
Loughborough University
Loughborough
Leicestershire
LE11 3TU
United Kingdom
E-mail: k.tolfrey@lboro.ac.uk

A. Tonson
Center for Magnetic Resonance in
Biology and Medicine (CRMBM)
UMR CNRS 6612
Medical School of Marseille
27, Bd Jean Moulin
13385 Marseille cedex 05
France
E-mail: anne.tonson@univmed.fr

A. Tremblay
Departement of Social and
Preventive Medicine
University of Laval
Quebec
Canada
E-mail:
angelo.tremblay@kin.msp.ulaval.ca

M.S. Tremblay
Healthy Active Living and Obesity
Research (HALO)
Department of Pediatrics, University
of Ottawa
CHEO Research Institute
401 Smyth Road
Ottawa, ON
K1H 8L1
Canada
E-mail: mtremblay@cheo.on.ca

M. Uvacsek
Semmelweis University Budapest
1123 Alkotas str. 44
Hungary
E-mail: martina@mail.hupe.hu

M. Van Brussel
Department of Pediatric
Physiotherapy and Exercise
Physiology
Wilhelmina Children's Hospital
University Medical Center Utrecht
Room KB2.056.0
PO Box 85090
3508 AB Utrecht
the Netherlands
E-mail:
m.vanbrussel@umcutrecht.nl

E. Van Praagh
Laboratory of Exercise Biology,
Clermont-Ferrand II
Bâtiment de Biologie B
Campus des Cézeaux
63177 Aubière
France
E-mail:
emmanuel.vanpraagh@wanadoo.fr

O. Verschuren
Centre of Excellence Rehabilitation
Centre 'De Hoogstraat'
Rembrandtkade 10
3583 TM Utrecht
The Netherlands
E-mail:
o.verschuren@dehoogstraat.nl

R.J. Willcocks
Children's Health and Exercise
Research Centre
School of Sport and Health Science
University of Exeter
Exeter, United Kingdom
EX1 2LQ
E-mail: rw254@exeter.ac.uk

C.A. Williams
School of Sport and Health Sciences
University of Exeter
United Kingdom
E-mail C.A.Williams@exeter.ac.uk

Author Index

General Index